Donated

FAT

ABOUT THE AUTHOR

Lisa Colles is a broadcast and print journalist, and is associate producer of the *FAT* television series. She lives in London.

THIS IS A CARLTON BOOK

Text Copyright © Carlton Television Ltd 1998
Design Copyright © Carlton Books Ltd 1998

First published in 1998 by Carlton Books Limited

A CIP catalogue record for this book is available from the British Library

ISBN 1 85868 580 X

Printed and bound in Great Britain

This book accompanies the ITV documentary series written, produced
and directed by Antony Thomas.

FAT

Exploding the Myths

LISA COLLES

CARLTON

**To Mum,
for your love and wisdom**

Contents

The Pima Indians, What is Obesity?, Our Toxic Food Environment, Tricks of the Trade, Warning: This Food Could Kill, Our Sedentary Lives, The Western Takeover, Getting Activated.

Back to the Pima Indians, Genetic Research, Metabolic Research, Big, Bad Seductive Fat, The Non-Fat Fat, Low-Fat Foods.

The Playground Effect, The Dieting Generation, Liposuction, On the Catwalk, Eating Disorders, Anorexia, The Rhodes Farm Day, Meal Times, Rhodes Farm Clinic: Patients' Stories, Bulimia, Who Sets the 'Ideal'?

Acknowledgements

Firstly, my thanks to Antony Thomas; for your help, and for the opportunity of working on the series, I thank you. Thanks also to the entire *FAT* team: Jonathan Partridge, Simon Farmer, Michael O'Donohue, Carleen Hsu, Brian Robertshaw, John Valadez and Sophie Todd. Many thanks to Dr Andrew Prentice for invaluable assistance and advice. At Carlton Television my thanks to Sian Facer, Don Christopher, Ruth Willows, Brendan Mannix, and Julie Stoner for so much help and support, and at Carlton Books my gratitude to Julian Flanders, Piers Murray Hill and May Corlfield. For words of wisdom and encouragement I am eternally grateful to Oonah Newbury, Adam Courtenay, Gavin Allen, Jane Cameron, Pippa Healy, Janice Rowe, Peter McHugh, and Rosanna Guneratne. My love to Anthony Boxshall for being, well, Anth, and to Connie Woolston for being such an inspiration. For such delightful stress relief I'm indebted to Jacquie, Simon & Matthew Weedon. Thanks also to my family and to Barry Harnel and Mike McCurry, who may never know their influence. Finally, my sincere appreciation to everyone who took part in the series and this book.

Foreword by
Dr Andrew Prentice

It is said that every picture tells a story. But no picture of a fat person can hope to convey the complex way in which modern society views those who carry excess weight. Tragically the picture will be unable to do anything but trigger our ingrained prejudices however hard we try to suppress them.

A truer story is told here in the words of fat people and very fat people, and of the doctors and psychologists who try to help them. Their innermost thoughts have been recorded by award-winning director, Antony Thomas, and associate producer Lisa Colles, in the course of their detailed groundwork for the major new television series and this book that accompanies it.

This book takes an oblique view of an important issue and provides a fresh and ground-breaking perspective. It is the full spectrum of views from patient to expert which makes this book and the series so enlightening. At times heart-wrenching, at others controversial, it will almost certainly change your views on how medicine and society should respond to the current epidemic of obesity.

Dr Andrew Prentice,
Head of Energy Metabolism,
Dunn Clinical Nutrition Centre,
Cambridge

The Weight Loss War

'There was something different about my body from the very beginning. I was put on my first diet when I was just three weeks old because my mother thought I was getting fat. She was overweight and wanted me to avoid all the heartache she'd been though. I learned from my parents very early on that the world discriminates against fat people and that if I didn't want my opportunities to be severely limited, I needed to lose weight.

'When I was about six I was started on amphetamine slimming pills. Pictures taken of me at that time show me looking really happy. The truth is I was very stoned. I'd spend my time running around the house trying desperately to get rid of that feeling you have when you're speeding. By the time I was 10 I still hadn't lost any weight, and I was already really scared about how I would cope as a fat teenager. How could I go to junior high school and take the kind of abuse I knew I would get?

'At 15 I went on my really big diet. That was when I started taking the amphetamine-like slimming drug phentermine, and I took a lot of it. You develop a tolerance to it and you have to take more and more to get the same effect. I was really speeding and I was using up prescriptions like crazy but the doctor just kept giving them to me; after all, the most important thing was that I got thin. It didn't matter that I was dizzy and hooked on the pills. He used to say to me, "We'll just worry about that when you're thin". So I ate two hard-boiled eggs a day and two stalks of celery, and I became totally obsessed with food.

'I did everything I had to do to try and lose weight and keep it off, but without success. The weight kept piling on, and I took it as a personal failure. I wasn't good enough. If only I could stop eating forever and keep the weight off; no matter what I did though, it always came back. It was after all this dieting, I believe, that my metabolism got so screwed up. In order to lose weight I had to eat well under 500 calories a day. If I ate over 1,000 calories a day I could gain a full pound in a day, and believe me I knew, because I kept very close track of what I ate.

'By the age of 22 I weighed about 235 pounds. I got desperate. I went to a therapist, because I thought there must be something wrong with me, but it didn't help. Every day I would get up and say, "Okay, I'm going to start a diet today", just as I had hundreds of times before. But I just couldn't do it any more. I never actually made a decision to stop dieting; my body just wouldn't let me be that cruel to myself again. I'm now 48, and since that time I've really begun to understand the part dieting played in my life and my relationship to food. I've been working out who I am as a person, and trying to undo the enormous amount of damage that was done to me as a dieting child.

'I never knew when I was hungry and when I wasn't; I never learned those cues. I eat more than most people, absolutely, it would be really bizarre if I didn't. But do I technically eat enough on a day to day basis that I should be this size? Probably not. A lot of my weight, I believe, is to do with genetics and the damage done to me by dieting. Had I not dieted and taken pills, I am convinced I would not be the 500 pound woman I am now. I might be 300 pounds, and there's a very big difference. I know what it feels like to be smaller; to get to be 500 pounds you start at zero and go through every single pound in between. When I was 300, even 400 pounds I could still dance all night. Now I can't do that.

'I have looked at everything in the search for a way to lose weight. But I believe there is nothing out there. I would never want to be a thin person – I like fat bodies aesthetically – but yes, if there was something out there that could help me lose 100 or 200 pounds, I would have done it, trust me. I do have a lot of limitations with my body. It's absolutely true that I consider myself disabled by my size. I can't sit in a chair all day because it's not comfortable and walking is very problematic for me. But what's really horrible for me is the way I'm treated in society; it's so much worse than anything else I have to deal with.

'I have suffered harassment from a very young age. I have a vivid memory of being five or six years old and walking through a park, with boys on bicycles surrounding me and trying to make me run. I've had people try to run me down in cars. It's always there, and the fatter you are the worse it is. People feel they have permission to be so invasive towards you and to make assumptions about you. Total strangers have come up to me and taken my food away. We fat people have to get angry. I think it's the only appropriate response to what has been done to us. And I think it's important for me to talk about my experiences because I really am the worst-case scenario. I am what everybody is afraid of becoming.

'But despite all this, I have felt comfortable with my body for many years now. It's funny because I cannot maintain weight ever; I'm always climbing very slowly no matter what I eat. Learning to love your body is a skill, and although it is difficult to be in a super-sized body, it is the body that I have. It's what's been given to me and I try to work with it and feel good about myself. That's really the best that I can do, and feeling good about ourselves is what we all deserve.

'I've had to learn how to exercise for the sheer joy of moving my body, and that has meant having to display myself and letting people see my belly move and my arms move, and that's probably the hardest thing I've done in my life so far. But I really love exercise, because it's part of loving my body. It's taken a long time, but I have learned to really appreciate what's different about my body, and how it looks and moves, and to really understand that it's not better and not worse than anyone else's; it's just different, and there's a beauty in difference. And this feels wonderful. It's the most freeing thing in the world. I feel that I have liberated myself from the prison I was in, and I'm never going back.'

Lynn McAfee

Measurements and Abbreviations

CLOTHES SIZES

The table below shows standard UK clothing sizes alongside their US equivalents:

UK size	US size
8	6
10	8
12	10
14	12
16	14
18	16
20	18
22	20
24	22
26	24
28	26
30	28

ABBREVIATIONS

For the convenience of the reader the following abbreviations for weights and measures have been used throughout the text:
Ounces: oz.
Pounds: lb.
Stones: st.
Feet: ft.
Inches: in.
Litres: l.
Kilograms: kg.
Calories: cal.

Introduction

Never has the immense, controversial and emotive subject that is FAT been more topical. In the Western world, and increasingly in the developing world, our intense preoccupation with body weight is expanding in direct proportion to our waistlines. In fact, according to some experts, we are in the midst of an 'obesity pandemic', a crisis so great the World Health Organisation was recently prompted to set up an Anti Obesity Task Force.

But what exactly is causing this crisis? Why, in the late 20th century when we are more body-obsessed than ever before, are we rapidly getting fatter? Is it the fault of the individual; a matter of greed and poor self-control? Or is society to blame, luring us into sedentary lives and seducing us with, as one expert terms it, a 'toxic food environment'. What about genes? Is body size inherited, as height and hair colour are inherited?

The irony is that we are getting fatter at a time when multi-billion pound markets in diet programmes, health clubs and low-fat foods are booming. In addition, it seems we are being pulled in opposite directions by two powerful, conflicting forces. On one hand, we're constantly exposed to the message that we must be thin to be attractive, successful and desirable; on the other, we're bombarded with seductive images of delicious, fattening, cheap food; everywhere we go advertisers tempt us to eat, eat, eat. The suggestion is, 'Eat everything, but don't you dare get fat'.

But what if we do get fat? Just how easy is it to lose weight and keep it off? Do diet programmes work, or, as a recent study has suggested, do 95 per cent of people who lose weight gain it all back – and often more – within five years? Is there any weight loss method guaranteed to succeed in the long term? Do low-fat foods help, or simply encourage consumers to eat more? And will scientists ever find the 'magic bullet' they are looking for – the pill that will melt away fat with neither risk nor effort?

But do we even need to worry about our weight? Some experts say it is perfectly possible to be fat, fit and healthy, and that there is a broad spectrum of ideal weights for each individual. So does it matter if a person is a few pounds, or even a few stones, overweight? Is there a proven connection between weight and ill-health, or is it really vanity – the abstract belief that slim is beautiful – that drives many of us to count calories obsessively and pound on treadmills in pursuit of the 'ideal'?

And just who sets these standards? What role does the media play in making us dissatisfied with ourselves? Every day we are bombarded with images of the ideal, the ultra-thin supermodels, but what lengths do they actually go to to maintain their bodies? Is it even healthy to be that thin? Who says women should look like Kate Moss, when in Rubens' time, and as recently as the 1950s, voluptuous women were considered not only desirable but healthy? Why should the well-rounded body now have come to signify failure and self-neglect? Why does prejudice based on body size appear to be the last permitted form of discrimination? And in the midst of all this, is it ever possible to be overweight and happy?

What does it say about our society when all of these issues combine to drive four year old girls to diet because 'I look in the mirror and I hate my body'? Hundreds of thousands of people across the world are currently suffering from eating disorders like anorexia and bulimia – conditions that were virtually unheard of a generation ago. However, for every one of these cases, there are perhaps 50 others who have lost their private battle against fat and are now far, far beyond the weight of their dreams.

The truth is, there is scarcely a man or woman out there who has not worried about their weight at some time during their lives. A recent British survey revealed that 45 per cent of children between the ages of 11 and 15 have already begun to worry about their weight, while American researchers have come up with another alarming statistic: 80 per cent of the nation's women dislike their own bodies.

Fat: Exploding the Myths sets out to explore all sides of this complex and controversial subject, and to provide answers for the many questions raised. In the course of researching the series and the book, we have interviewed over 100 international experts in the field, along the way gaining access to the latest research. We have been to slimming clinics, gyms, hospitals, schools, universities, eating disorders clinics, obesity clinics, fashion shows and magazines, food manufacturing companies, 'fat acceptance' groups and private homes where we have met hundreds of people whose lives and careers are dominated by fat. *Fat: Exploding the Myths* brings their stories to life.

CHAPTER ONE

THE FAT TRAP

'The average American child sees 10,000 advertisements each year on television alone. Ninety-five per cent of those are for one of four types of foods: fast foods, soft drinks, sugar-coated cereals and candy. And that's 10,000 messages by the brightest minds in advertising that convince children to eat foods that are bad for them.'

Kelly Brownell, Professor of Psychology,
Epidemiology & Public Health, Yale University

The statistics are stark. The Department of Health *Health Survey for England* published in January 1998 discovered that 16 per cent of men and 17 per cent of women in England are obese. In addition to this, 45 per cent men and 34 per cent of women are considered overweight. And on the other side of the Atlantic things are even worse. One third of the adult population in the US is obese, with the figure rising to 50 per cent in some ethnic groupings, and by some estimates as many as 30 per cent of American children are over-weight. Indeed, the average person in the US gains about 1lb. in weight a year after the age of 25; that's a 30lb. gain by the age of 55. One study estimates that the entire population of America will be obese by 2230.

Just what is it about life in the late 20th century that is causing us to lose control so dramatically?

The Pima Indians

Twenty miles south of Phoenix, Arizona, the Casa Blanca Road skirts the border of the Gila River Indian Community, home to a tribe of American Indians called the Pima. Their ancestors split into two groups during the Middle Ages, one settling here in Arizona and the other migrating to an area known as Maycoba, in Mexico. Genetically, the two tribes are almost identical, but there is one characteristic in which they differ dramatically. The Mexican Pima are an average of 57lb. lighter than their Arizona cousins.

In the early 1900s, the Arizona Pima were forced to stop their traditional farming when white settlers diverted the upper waters of the Gila River; the Pima's irrigation canals ran dry and the land died. For more than half a century, the Pima here were reduced to dependency, barely keeping alive on government subsidy. Many suffered from poverty, malnutrition and even starvation. Then, in 1984, their fortunes changed. The Pima were granted a casino concession in the heart of this prosperous American state where gambling is otherwise forbidden. On a good day, bus loads of visitors flock here and blow away thousands upon thousands of dollars.

Profits now pour into community coffers, but above all, the casino offers the Pima Indians opportunities to work as managers, security staff, cleaners, cooks, croupiers and drivers. They are now well and truly back in business; the links to their ancestral land broken, the Pima have joined the American mainstream. Today this Arizona tribe shares the American culture, the American lifestyle, and the American diet. Fast foods are widely available to them and their diet, like that of other Americans, contains about 40 per cent fat. In one respect, however, they have outdone their fellow Americans. They are now the fattest population group in the United States.

In the reservation's Hu Hu Kam Memorial Hospital, funded by casino profits, the Pima Indians cope with diseases linked to obesity – hypertension, high blood pressure, several forms of cancer, bone, joint and muscle strains, sleep apnoea and diabetes. A . per cent of adult Pimas in the community are diabetic, . cent of those with diabetes are overweight. A dialysis clin. ates 14 hours a day, six days a week, treating three groups patients each day. In this hospital they are proud, and rightly so, of their achievements. No one pays for treatment and the whole population is carefully monitored. The Pima have also allowed the American government to use their hospital as a human laboratory. Two thousand Pima volunteers undergo regular testing in an important long-term study of obesity and diabetes for the American National Institute of Health.

Four hundred miles to the south, however, high in the Sierra Madre mountains of Northern Mexico, an isolated Pima Indian community of just 700 people continues to live a traditional life off the land, as subsistence farmers. They eat a diet consisting largely of grains, fruits and vegetables, as their ancestors have for centuries; in total they eat about half as much as the Arizona Pima. Each week they engage in over 20 hours of hard physical labour, ploughing and tending to their crops and their animals, carrying water, building shelter and doing anything else they need to survive; the Pima in Arizona average two hours of physical activity per week. The Mexican Pima have no labour-saving devices, not even electricity or piped water; they are generally fit, lean and healthy.

The Mexican Pima provide us with a graphic example of the way our environment and lifestyle can influence our weight and health. And in the Western world in particular, it seems, our environment is spinning out of control.

What is Obesity?

People are considered to be overweight or obese when they have excess body fat. But what exactly is excess? The medical profession has developed the Body Mass Index (BMI), which is used for calculating levels of overweight. Someone with a BMI of over 30 is considered obese: that is more than 20 percent over their 'ideal'.

$$\text{BMI} = \frac{\text{Weight(Kg)}}{\text{Height x Height(m)}}$$

In order to make BMI measurements more easily understood, a grading system has been developed, as follows:

Grade of obesity	BMI	Description
Grade 0	20 - 24.9	Desirable weight
Grade 1	25 - 29.9	Overweight
Grade 2	30 - 40	Obese
Grade 3	> 40	Severely/ mordidly obese

Even with the grading system, it is still difficult to visualize exactly what a BMI of a certain value actually means, and the effects that weight gain has on BMI.

For example
1) A person of 5ft. 2in. (1.58m), weighing 15st. 10lb. (100kg) has a BMI of 40 and would be classified as being severely obese. To achieve a BMI of 25 (the upper cut off for desirable weight) a weight loss of nearly 6st (37.6kg) would be needed.

2) A person of 6ft. (1.83m), weighing 13st. (82.55kg) has a BMI of 24.75 and would be classified as being of a desirable weight. However, if this individual gained 1st., making them 14st. (89kg), their BMI would change to 26.60, which is classified as overweight.

The following graph makes working out BMI even easier:

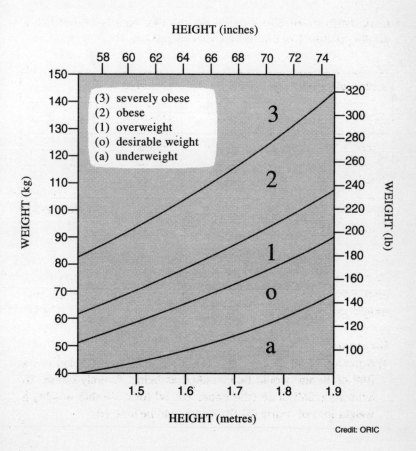

HEIGHT (inches)

WEIGHT (kg)

(3) severely obese
(2) obese
(1) overweight
(o) desirable weight
(a) underweight

WEIGHT (lb)

HEIGHT (metres)

Credit: ORIC

Our Toxic Food Environment

Professor Kelly Brownell is a man with a mission. As Professor of Psychology, Epidemiology & Public Health at Yale University and Director of the Yale Centre for Eating & Weight Disorders, Brownell has spent more than 20 years researching, among other things, weight gain, obesity and the environment.

'There really is a global epidemic of obesity,' he states. 'The problem is most pronounced in the United States, but other developed countries are catching up, and we're seeing more and more obesity in countries that were undeveloped and are now becoming more Westernized.' And obesity, he says, carries a terrible toll. 'There's the emotional suffering of people who have obesity and there's also a terrible health toll. And the numbers are getting so large that it really should be considered an epidemic. Some serious steps need to be taken.' However, Brownell points out, this is a very complex issue. 'This is a field where there are multiple, powerful collisions between different points of view and different forces, acting in different directions.' On one hand, for example, is the need to keep body weight in perspective, and not have people crazed and trying to look a way they never can. 'On the other hand, we do have this epidemic that's spiralling out of control, and nowhere is it more clear than in the US, with Britain catching up.'

Brownell says there are three logical places to look in trying to work out who or what is to blame for this epidemic. One is with the individual, he says, and the idea that people are making bad choices, are lacking will-power and doing something wrong in their lives which leads them to overeat and not exercise enough. 'This is where society has been laying the blame for decade after decade. All the weight loss programmes are based on this assumption that people are doing something wrong; if they come to the programme and they correct it, they should get better,' he says. The problem with this approach, Brownell explains, is that, 'blaming the victim is not very productive. We're not doing anything about the epidemic of obesity despite all these weight loss programmes focused on the individual and blaming the victim.' In fact, he points out, the problem just continues to get worse.

'The second logical place to look is biology, and genetics in particular. Genetics permit obesity, but they don't cause it,' says Brownell. 'You cannot attribute the 25 per cent increase in the prevalence of obesity in the United States in the past 10 years to a change in the genetic pool.' Genes simply do not evolve that quickly. 'The cause,' he states, 'is the toxic food environment. Unlike any society in the history of the world, we now have available to us "poor" foods, they're widely available, heavily promoted and are available at low cost so that they're accessible to all segments of society. And as long as these foods are there and people enjoy eating them, because they also tend to taste very good, we're going to have problems with obesity.'

Tricks of the Trade

The environment we live in has grown progressively more toxic over the past 10 or 20 years, says Brownell. 'One can see in country after country after country that if the environment gets more modernised and more Westernized, the prevalence of obesity increases. If we're going to intervene and do something about the epidemic, we need to change the environment.' High-fat, high-calorie foods are all around us, says Brownell. The toxic environment comes at us from many angles, and the access to high-fat, high-calorie foods is very widespread; it comes in supermarkets with their rows and rows of highly processed, attractively packaged, high-fat foods. 'It comes in fast-food restaurants like McDonald's and Burger King, it comes in little mini-markets and service stations, and it even comes in schools,' says Brownell. 'There are places in the United States where there are fast food franchises right inside schools, and sometimes even inside children's hospitals. And so the infiltration of poor food into the environment is nearly complete.'

And with these type of foods so heavily advertised and promoted, Brownell says it's no wonder so many people have a hard time resisting them, though children are particularly vulnerable. 'The average American child sees 10,000 commercials for food advertised a year on television alone, and 95 per cent of those are for one of four different types of foods: fast food, soft drinks, sugar coated cereals or candy. And that's 10,000 messages made by the brightest minds in advertising that convince children to eat foods that are bad for them.'

Brownell explains that advertisers use all sorts of tricks to sell food products, and to make them appear healthy when they simply are not. 'Many of their practices are deceptive. For example when a sugar-coated cereal that could be half its weight in sugar is advertised, it might be shown surrounded by healthy foods like fruit and a glass of milk or a piece of toast,' he says, 'and they'll make out that this cereal is part of a nutritious breakfast. In fact that's a line American children recognize, "part of this nutritious breakfast", the implication being that you can eat this cereal that doesn't have much nutrition and has an awful lot of sugar, and be healthy in doing so.

'Advertisers are very creative,' Brownell continues, 'and the blitz of advertising that occurs is very impressive. And while it's true that there's free choice and that parents have a responsibility to educate their children, the fact is that parents are exposed to the same advertising their children are.' As a result, Brownell believes it's very hard for parents to counter those 10,000 messages that are so cleverly and persuasively done. 'And schools don't have time to do nutrition education, so what children learn about food is mainly via television and through what their parents serve them. 'We are raising generation after generation of children who are learning to eat foods that are just not good for them. They're learning to eat large serving sizes, they're learning to eat beyond the point where they're physically full, they're learning to eat to feel psychologically gratified, and as a consequence we have this epidemic of obesity that I predict will continue to grow worse.'

Brownell also sees fast food restaurants as particularly culpable. 'Any nutritionist will tell you that a meal that is laden with calories and fat and salt is not good for you, and that's what most fast foods contain. Having said that, you could go into a restaurant like McDonald's and, if you were crafty, put together a reasonable meal. But most people don't do that. They want the Big Macs and quarter pounders with cheese, the large French fries and the soft drinks, milk shakes and so on, and if people eat enough of those foods it's going to be unhealthy for them.

Food Labelling

Fast food manufacturers often claim that if customers want to know more about what's in their food, they have nutritional information leaflets on offer, listing ingredient and nutrient contents. However, Professor Philip James, Director of Aberdeen's Rowett Research Institute, says these leaflets are in fact so complex they can really only be understood by analytical chemists. 'Not one in a hundred people can make an informed choice on the basis of this information. The fast-food people are constantly misleading with completely unintelligible labelling. It's all put into the wrong mode, deliberately. You would have to be a super-nutritionist like me and have a special computer and a machine to measure metabolic rate to have a hope-in-hell of interpreting the food labels in terms of energy balance,' he states. 'Food labelling really has nothing to do with consumer education or with helping people to choose an appropriate diet. It's a con,' he says.

'Food like this is very dense in calories and fat, but people are drawn to it because it tastes good and it's cheap. Of course the calories make people put on weight, and the fat leads to negative health problems' he says. 'There's nothing wrong with eating a Big Mac and fries once in a while, but the fact is that people eat them too much. On any one day, seven per cent of the American population will eat at McDonald's, and that is only one of a huge number of fast food restaurants and chains across the country. If you add all the others, the number just grows and grows,' he says.

'McDonald's boasts that it has served 99 billion people, so I ask you, is it good for the collective body of people in the modern environment that billions and billions of people have eaten those hamburgers and French fries and soft drinks? The answer is unquestionably no.' It's not good for us, he says, and so access to those foods has to be changed. 'McDonald's stated corporate goal is that no American should be more than four minutes from one of its outlets. The fact we view this as acceptable and tolerable is remarkable to me.'

Added to this, people are also being seduced by big portions and the idea that they are getting value for money. 'The serving sizes in many restaurants in the United States are enormous. People often bring food home with them from restaurants because their serving was too large,' Brownell says. 'And foods are packaged in ways that encourage people to eat more. Fast food restaurants offer what they call value meals, packaged meals where if you order a number of items together it will cost less than if you order them individually. You might get a big hamburger, a big order of fries and a large soft drink. If you put all those things together the collective impact in terms of sugar and fat and calories is enormous. In some cases, you're going to get about 900 calories from just the drink and the fries alone, and that's before you even touch the main feature of the meal, which could be something like a double cheeseburger with bacon.'

So, while people feel they're getting a good deal financially, according to Brownell they're not doing themselves any favours. 'If their goal is to pack as many calories and grams of fat into their body as is possible, then it would be a splendid deal, but in terms of health, the effect is negative.' Plus, not only are we being persuaded to eat foods that are bad for us, this is also teaching us to eat more than we actually need.

'We no longer give eating the attention it deserves. We tend not to sit down and enjoy our meals the way Europeans do. Instead we rush in and out and just grab food as sustenance before rushing on to the next overcrowded event... People aren't getting a balanced diet. They're not getting fruits and vegetables; they grab fried foods and too many high sugar, high fat foods, because these are the easiest and most available.'

Dr Janet Polivy, Department of Psychology, University of Toronto

Brownell points out that just 10 minutes away from his Yale office there is a section of road crammed with one fast food outlet after another, and that this is typical of what he terms the 'American food landscape'. 'If I drive down that road for just 10 minutes I pass about 30 different places where one could get highly processed, high-calorie, high-fat food. There are fast food restaurants that are open 24 hours, ones that have drive-through facilities so that you don't even have to get out of your car to get a meal, places that offer "all you can eat" buffets for an inclusive low price, service stations that have been remodelled with mini-markets inside, and all promoting high-fat food at low cost. This is what I call the toxic food environment, and it's my belief that we're poisoning ourselves with it.'

Warning: This Food Could Kill

Brownell has some radical suggestions about how we might conquer this toxic food environment. 'I believe that the first step in dealing with this environment is to develop a militant attitude, like we have with tobacco. As a culture we have decided to take action against the cigarette industry because so many people are dying from tobacco-related illnesses. We have intervened by regulating and legislating, so the use of tobacco goes down. We tax cigarettes, we ban smoking in offices and public places and we regulate advertising.

'In the United States about 500,000 deaths a year can be attributed to cigarette smoking, but now 300,000 deaths are related to poor diet,' he says, 'and I believe that with figures like that, we've reached a point where we need to take social action. Something bold needs to be done.' Brownell is campaigning for a four-point action plan to be put into place. 'Firstly I would seek to subsidize the sale of healthy foods, for example by cutting the cost of fruit and vegetables by 75 per cent so that people would have more access to them. In that way, healthier foods might displace the more unhealthy foods people are eating now.

'If that weren't sufficient to have a major public health impact, I would also consider raising the price of bad foods, perhaps by imposing some sort of tax, like we do on tobacco. If the cost of bad foods went up, maybe people would eat less of them. Then, I would intervene in the advertising of food, so that ads aimed at children were regulated like we regulate cigarette advertising aimed at children. Camel cigarettes use the image of Joe Camel, which many people feel encourages kids to smoke. McDonald's uses Ronald McDonald to encourage kids to eat food that is bad for them. I ask you, is there really a difference? Finally, I would provide opportunities for the population to be more physically active by building bike paths, recreation centres, and encouraging physical activity in schools.'

Some might argue that Brownell's ideas strike right at the heart of free market capitalism and consumers' freedom of choice, but the professor stresses this is not his wish. 'My first choice in dealing with the epidemic of obesity would be to turn responsibility over to individuals and hope they make the right choices, hope they get control over their eating and their exercise and their weight. In an ideal world we could rely on people to make the right choices in their lives so that we would have a healthy culture and a healthy environment.' But, Brownell says, the pressures on consumers are now so great that things have got out of hand. 'There comes a time where people aren't able to take responsibility, and taking social action seems to be justified.'

Brownell admits that the idea of controlling the toxic food environment is new, and that there are few other advocates of it at present. 'I think the problem will get worse before it gets better. As long as the bad food is out there in abundance, and it's heavily promoted and advertised, it tastes good and it's so widely available, we're going to have very bad problems with obesity.' But, he says, 'If you do nothing more than eat more fruit and vegetables and less junk food, you can go a long way towards eating a truly healthy diet.'

Our Sedentary Lives

'We have a totally global – I mean totally global – pandemic of obesity. It is hard to overstate the seriousness. You see it in all corners of the world. I am getting frightening data from China, Malaysia, Brazil. The whole thing is exploding.' These are the words of Professor Philip James, Director of Aberdeen's Rowett Research Institute. He has studied obesity and its impact for many years. 'The challenge for me and my colleagues is how we are going to convert the medical world and society to think in a very different way, because we can predict that every five to seven years we're likely to see a doubling in the obesity rate almost in any country in the world you care to look at. It is just the most nightmarish scenario.'

Like Professor Brownell, James agrees the problem lies in our environment. 'There has been a complete collapse in the amount of physical activity that children, young people and the ordinary adult has to do, and we've completely altered the everyday diet over the last 30 years.' And we have to remember, James says, that this change in physical activity and diet has never been seen before in the history of mankind. 'The fact is, in the post-war period, industry has done a brilliant job in answering the human demand to do less work. On trips to Ethiopia I have seen the energy cost, the agony of carrying water, of ploughing, of doing a whole host of things. It's painful, and you discover that the men and women just collapse at the end of the day. So, throughout history we've been attempting to devise ways so that we don't have to do so much work, and as a result the whole post-war period has been a glorious success story in terms of reducing the amount of physical activity we have to do.

'Now, I can just get in my car and go wherever I want, instantly. It's just the most addictive phenomenon. And this car culture has been promoted systematically by governments throughout the world, but it has had a huge effect on the amount of physical activity we do. Then, in comes television, which is also gloriously seductive. At long last it's possible to just sit, without having to read or even concentrate particularly, to just sit in front of a television, and people find it wonderful. But it's had a very powerful effect in terms of our engendering a completely sedentary lifestyle.'

And even our working lives have been revolutionized. 'Suddenly we don't have to walk around factories any more. Everything is computerized and mechanically organized, and instead of physically making things and standing on our feet all day, we now sit down at computers.' So, there has been a transformation in the way we move around, a complete revolution in the circumstances at work, and the seductive ability to just collapse in our chairs at home and watch a whole fascinating array of entertainment. 'These three things, I think, have completely transformed the amount of energy we use as part of our daily routines.'

Dr Andrew Prentice, Head of Energy Metabolism at the Dunn Clinical Nutrition Centre in Cambridge, agrees, but adds that this increasingly sedentary way of life has managed to creep up on us. 'It's an invidious, silent change which nobody notices. It's an enormous social change,' he says. 'We have moved to a society where everything is done for us by some gadget. If you stand at the bottom of an escalator on the London Underground, one with a staircase in the middle, you'll find enormous queues gathering at the bottom of the escalator and the stairs not being used. Doors open without us pushing them; there's power steering on cars and automatic locking that removes the need to walk round the car,' he says.

Add to this children being dropped off at school, automatic garage doors, dishwashers and washing machines, and drive-through banks and food outlets and the truth becomes even clearer. 'The cumulative effect of all these labour-saving devices is to reduce our energy expenditure in an incredible way, but also in a silent way. And television is the worst possible thing.' All these things, Prentice says, have made us so susceptible to weight gain. 'It is basically the environment and our behaviour that is making so many people become overweight. It is often pointed out that you never found a fat person in Belsen.' But, he adds, the forces working against us are tremendous.

'We have never spent more on technological devices to stop us spending energy, and we have never spent more on advertising high-fat, very palatable foods and developing new foods than we have at the moment.' And these factors, Prentice says, are fighting against all the millions of pounds people spend in trying to lose weight, and against the little that is spent on intelligent public health messages and health promotion campaigns.

The Western Takeover

All over the world, a similar transformation is taking place, and not just in the West. China, with its population of 1.2 billion people, has managed, until now, to remain relatively untouched by the developed world. But things are changing fast. Beijing is now a vast construction site. Foreign investors, lured by the prospect of a cheap, highly-competent labour force and a potential market of over a billion consumers, pour money into the country. The speed of change is dizzying. Bicycle traffic that only recently had command of the streets has now been squeezed into the margins; car ownership is rising at a rapid rate. Beijing has come to look like any successful capital city: brash, exciting, innovative, polluted and jammed solid.

In the back streets, vendors still ply delicious varieties of healthy, traditional Chinese food, but tastes are changing. The sudden release from conformity and control has created an insatiable appetite for anything new - and invariably that means anything Western. Today, the Chinese, and particularly the young, want everything we've got to offer. And, of course, we are always happy to sell it to them. Not long after the Tiananmen Square uprising, the McDonald's Corporation tentatively set up an outlet in Beijing. Very quickly all the main American food manufacturers and fast food chains joined in the rush to take a slice of this lucrative and expanding market.

There are now fast food restaurants on just about every street corner. McDonald's alone has 53 outlets in Beijing, and just as it does everywhere else, the Corporation directs its advertising at children. And in China, where parents are forbidden by law to have more than one child, this is a particularly rewarding strategy. The little emperors, as these precious 'only' children are called, are indulged. And now, China faces an epidemic of child-onset obesity dating, almost exactly, from the arrival of the American fast foods, soft drinks and confectionery. It is estimated that each year another 10 per cent of urban China's under seven-year-olds are classified as obese. One recent survey found that over 70 million Chinese people are overweight; many, many of these are children. And all this in a country that for centuries battled against famine. In fact, obesity was practically unheard of here a decade ago.

Now special clinics and summer camps – not unlike those in America – have been set up to treat these obese children. Beijing has several of these clinics. At one Professor Zhang treats about 1,000 obese children, almost all of them boys. Song Bo Wen, for example, is 12 years old and was a massive 16st. 7lb. when he first attended the clinic four months ago. Now he is proud to have dropped 4st., to 12st. 7lb. Zhang's prescriptions are conventional: appetite suppressants, a diet of lean meat, fruit, vegetables and massive doses of encouragement and exercise. But will this be enough to stem the growth of obesity in China, to fight the immense influence of the West? If the continued growth of obesity in the West despite all the diet programmes and products available is an indicator, the answer is a resounding no.

Getting Activated

Professor Philip James believes we've got ourselves into a mess of individual blame where overweight is concerned. He feels it is far too easy to say, 'It's your problem, you're at fault', to someone who is overweight, when actually the whole of society is no longer geared to allowing people to maintain a reasonable weight. 'Sometimes people who do manage to keep their weight down will imply very confidently that they're superior beings, that they've got complete control. And really they're often simply genetically lucky, and perhaps they happen to have been brought up in an environment where they've been quite active, but they claim it as a special attribute.

'We've got to change the whole way in which we behave as a society. We've got to put people into an environment where they're naturally physically active. The wonderful thing to do is just be on your feet, wandering around or ideally walking so that you add about an hour's walking a day,' he says. And as well as this we have to change the whole nature of the foods we eat. 'We have to recognize that these wonderfully processed foods that are energy packed are no good, and we need to develop a whole array of delightful vegetable, plant-based foods that are not stacked with fats and sugars.' In short, he says, we're going to have to change the whole way in which we live and work. This sounds like a very tall order indeed.

James says countries like Norway and the Netherlands are slowly changing their environment. 'Take Norway for example. They have changed society so that it is normal for people to be pretty active, and they've dropped the fat content of the diet from 42 to 34 per cent, which is quite dramatic.' These changes can be achieved by encouraging people to use their cars less, to ride bikes or walk instead, for example. Many companies provide showers and changing rooms to encourage people to do just this, and public education campaigns promote healthy eating. In contrast, a recent US study found that in 1992 the National Cancer Institute spent $400,000 on a campaign to encourage the eating of more fruit and vegetables. That year, one cereal manufacturer spent an estimated $32 million to advertise just one product – sugar-frosted flakes.

The bottom line, says Dr Andrew Prentice, is that we have to educate people. 'And particularly educate youngsters and try and stop them getting into this terrible bind we ourselves have got into. We've got to teach them it's not their fault they're getting fat, that this is an environment humans have never seen before in the whole of their evolution,' And, he says, we need to explain what this environment is doing to people. 'We are now able to live almost without lifting a finger and this has an enormous effect on health and body weight regulation. We are seduced by enormous periods sat in front of the television,' he adds, 'and there's food about us the whole time which is tempting us to eat when we're not really hungry; never before has food been as cheap and as readily available.

'If we can teach people that it's the environment that is leading them astray, and give them the skills to protect themselves against this, then I think we can move forward.' People need to learn to live within a completely new set of environmental conditions. Prentice admits, however, that getting this message across and teaching people new ways to live will probably be difficult and expensive. 'That's why there is such a debate about whether we actually need to take this out of people's hands and do some fairly draconian things, like fat taxes' he says. 'Or, for instance, changing transport policy, making sure it's safe for children to play in the streets and getting physical activity into the school curriculum.'

With Professor Kelly Brownell's suggestions added to this list, there is clearly a lot of work to do. And it needs to be done soon. 'If we don't begin to start sorting this out now, we're going to be in enormous trouble because it's going to take 20 or 30 years to really begin to turn the tide,' warns Professor James.

CHAPTER TWO

GENES, METABOLISM & THE GLORY OF FAT

'Our obesity is in our stars. Our size is genetically determined. My eye colour is like that of my forebears. My hair or lack thereof is a genetic endowment, my uncle, my father, other individuals in my lineage were the same. The same with the breadth of shoulders, the length of my femur, the size of my feet, my ears, my nose. We all see that. We look at people and say, "Boy, that person looks like their father, mother, sister, brother," whatever. Us guys, we have a bigger belly; that's a genetic thing. Women, they have a bigger butt, bigger thighs. These are endowments that we all agree are genetic, even to the distribution of fat.

'There's only one thing left that people somehow do not accept as genetic. Every other measurement is accepted as inherited except the amount of weight. Now isn't that ridiculous? And today, there is no obesity geneticist that I know of in the world who does not agree that there is a genetic component in the cause of obesity... And if you have a predisposition to be large in your genes, and you're in the richest country in the world, you're going to be large. Because we live in a toxic food environment.'

Dr George Cowan, Obesity Surgeon,
University of Tennessee, Memphis

Back to the Pima Indians

As we have seen, the Pima Indians in Mexico are lean and fit, while their almost genetically identical Arizona cousins are largely obese. Their very different ways of life obviously play an important role in determining their body weights, but experts agree there is something else at play here. It seems that the Pima Indians have a genetic susceptibility for gaining weight easily. This is an example of what scientists call the 'thrifty gene' theory.

For thousands of years the Pima, while living and working off the land, have managed to survive seasonal highs and lows. That is, they have lived though times when food is available in abundance and then through times of great scarcity, such as between harvests or when crops have failed. As a result their genes have evolved and adapted so that when food is plentiful they put weight on easily, giving them a greater chance of survival, by living off stored body fat, when food is scarce. The problem for the Arizona Pima is that lack of food is no longer an issue. In fact, like most of the Western world, and in many developing countries, high-fat, high-calorie foods are available to them all the time. This, combined with lack of exercise, makes them far more susceptible to obesity than the population at large.

While their Mexican cousins continue to reap the rewards of their 'thrifty' genes, the Arizona Pima, in these modern times, don't stand a chance. They were not designed, genetically, for a world like the one we inhabit today. So in a sense, their weight is in their genes. But the fact is, it is only through being exposed to the modern environment – the toxic food environment and sedentary lifestyle – that this genetic predisposition causes problems; the genes are there, but it's exposure to the environment that causes obesity. The Mexican Pima, so long as they continue to live a traditional life, are very unlikely to become obese.

Genetic Research

One of the people at the forefront of research into the genetics of obesity is Dr Rudy Leibel, Professor of Paediatrics & Medicine and Principal Investigator in the Division of Molecular Genetics at New York's Columbia University. He believes that our genes play a role in determining how much body fat we have, but, he says, 'I think those genetic influences are very strongly influenced by the environment, and the circumstances in which an individual lives.' However, Leibel acknowledges that people are often intolerant of the idea that weight has anything to do with genes at all. 'If we went out on the street right now and looked at the people walking by, we would appreciate that there are ranges of height that might easily differ by as much as two and a half feet.' And if people were stopped and asked why differences in height occur, he says, most would give an answer related to genetics. 'It's in the family' for example.

'But, if we stopped a group of people on the street and said, "Why do you think you weigh less or more than the people walking next to you?", there would be all sorts of explanations, but very little to do with genes or genetic influences.' Leibel says explanations would probably range from, 'That person can't control their diet' and, 'That person's irresponsible', to the use of words like lazy and slothful. His belief, however, is that our weight is actually determined by far more complex factors. 'There are equally potent genetic influences on body weight as there are on height,' he states. 'But the population, because of our lack of understanding of all the mechanisms, has not come to accept this yet, so body weight is seen as, "Your problem, your fault, your personal and sole responsibility".'

This assumption, made by many, that people choose to eat their way into massive degrees of obesity is wrong, Leibel says. 'My argument is that the variations in body weight that we see out there on the street are strongly influenced by genetic factors.' He says we should no more blame individuals for their body weight – at least in the obese – than we should for their height.

Leibel and his colleagues have conducted experiments on mice, and found several genes that, when impaired, appear to cause obesity. One of these genes is responsible for the production of a hormone known as leptin, which is produced by the fat cells. Mice with a mutation in this gene have been shown to produce either no leptin, or a malformed version of it, and as a result grow to about three times their normal weight. Other hormones have been found to interact with leptin, and when working properly these reduce appetite and raise the metabolism after eating.

'The disorder of these genes produces a stronger pressure to eat and also a greater efficiency of metabolism, so that the animals get fat, both because they are hungrier and because the body spends less energy,' explains Leibel. 'These genes, therefore, are clearly very important in the normal regulation of the storage of body fat, because when they are disordered or mutant, they produce this rather striking change in behaviour; precisely the same sorts of behaviour that are seen in humans prior to the development of their own obesity.' In fact, researchers have found rare instances of gene defects in humans that appear to produce obesity which is similar to that seen in animals.

There is, however, still a long way to go before scientists really understand how these genes and hormones interact and work in humans. 'These genes are giving us access to brain chemicals that clearly play a very, very important part in weight regulation, both in animals and in humans,' says Leibel. 'My best hope is to be able to use the insights provided by the animals to design very effective and very highly targeted therapies to treat the problem in humans.' In fact, Leibel hopes that one day, it may be possible to replace mutant genes in humans. 'We now know there are very rare instances in which human obesity is due virtually entirely to the inappropriate function of a specific gene,' he says, adding that only three or four of these extreme cases have been found. 'I think in these very rare instances, it will ultimately be possible to correct the abnormality simply by the replacement of a single gene, as we have done with animals,' he says. However, Leibel feels that, after more research, human obesity will be found to be more commonly due to the malfunction, or slightly disordered function, of a series of genes. Replacing a series of genes will be far more difficult, he says.

Leibel and his team have also carried out research into how some people manage to maintain relatively constant body weight, whether that be slender people maintaining a lower body weight or obese people who, over a lifetime, remain obese. 'We have found evidence that there are very strong regulatory mechanisms in the body,' he explains. 'These mechanisms maintain you at the weight you were intended to be at, genetically and environmentally.' This, he says, is called the body's 'set point'. 'We have compared the metabolic response of an obese person undergoing a 10 per cent weight reduction to that of a normal weight individual undergoing a 10 per cent weight reduction, and found that the two individuals responded in precisely the same way to the loss in body weight. And that is', Leibel explains, 'that the body resists being deformed or pulled away from its usual body weight to a lower body weight. It resists this by increasing the drive to get food and by lowering the rate at which the body spends energy.'

And by lowering the metabolic rate so that less energy is used up, weight can be more easily regained. Basically, Leibel says, an obese person brought down to what looks like a more normal body weight is in fact in a metabolic state which very closely resembles that of starvation in a normal weight person. He points out that someone in this state of starvation suffers constant hunger and the drive to eat more, a sense of being cold and deprived and often depressed. 'It's a very difficult circumstance to place someone in and the vast majority of normal weight individuals couldn't tolerate those symptoms. And yet', Leibel says, 'it's felt that obese people should be asked to do this as a more or less routine consequence of weight reduction.' And Leibel believes this is why it is so difficult for some people to lose weight and maintain the loss. Once people lose weight, their metabolism slows down. 'They've actually been brought into a metabolic state which is abnormal for them.'

But Leibel acknowledges that whatever influence genes actually have, weight gain is the result of many factors. The amount of body fat people have, he says, is influenced by both genetic factors and the environment they live in. 'I don't think it's possible to separate the effect of the environment from genetic influences in most instances, and that's what makes this such a very complicated medical and social problem.'

Metabolic Research

Doctors Andrew Prentice and Susan Jebb of the Dunn Clinical Nutrition Centre in Cambridge have also been studying the effects of metabolism, weight regulation and fat in the diet for many years. 'Research in this area started about 20 years ago when I first moved into the field of energy metabolism, and everyone was of the view that, "It's my metabolism that's causing the problem, doctor". All I can say is that after hundreds of millions of dollars of research worldwide, we've failed to track down a single individual in whom there is persuasive evidence that they've got an abnormally low metabolic rate.'

During extensive studies, Prentice and his colleagues have put people though repeated cycles of weight loss and weight gain – as happens in yo-yo dieting – to see if this has a permanent effect on the metabolism. 'There is absolutely no doubt that metabolic rate goes down when we diet,' Prentice says. This action is evolutionary, it's the body's way of fighting back when it thinks it faces starvation, as Dr Leibel points out. 'But we have found that the metabolic rate recovers once given sufficient time, usually within a few weeks,' explains Prentice.

His colleague Dr Jebb explains that overweight people actually have higher metabolic rates than leaner people. 'It's quite clearly not the case that overweight people have slow metabolisms.' She explains this using the car as an analogy. 'If you've got the ignition turned on you will be using petrol, even if you're not going anywhere. And if you're in a big car with a two-litre engine, you'll be using far more energy than a small car with a one-litre engine,' she says. 'Quite simply, bigger people take more energy just to keep them going, to keep them ticking over even when they're not moving at all. And of course, when we look at physical activity, the bigger you are the more energy every single activity takes.'

However, Jebb explains that there are a range of metabolic processes which should keep the body in what is termed 'energy balance', but that these systems appear to be impaired in some people. 'For example, when we gain weight the metabolic rate increases,' she says, and that should act to bring the body back to somewhere near it's original weight or 'energy balance'. In some people however, this doesn't happen. 'Something more powerful is actually allowing weight gain to continue,' she explains. 'And at the moment, we haven't got to the bottom of that.' Dr Prentice adds that there is a huge debate as to whether the body has a 'set point'. 'The body does try to regulate its weight and fat balance over time,' he says, which indicates to him that there is a rough set point. But increasingly, in our modern world, this system of regulation is being sent askew.

Jebb, Prentice and their colleagues are doing a great deal of research into this question of why some people maintain their weight and others simply continue to get fatter. 'We're interested in how the body regulates its weight and fat balance over time. What are the basic processes that allow that to occur?' asks Prentice. 'What we know is that the system gets misled much more easily in some people than others. Why do some people simply go haywire when put into conditions of a high-fat diet and low physical activity?' Prentice says these 'twin evils', the hugely abundant food supply and enormous change in levels of physical activity, are confusing this system in so many people, causing many to succumb to overweight and obesity.

Prentice and Jebb use 'whole body calorimeters' to undertake their studies. These are carefully controlled rooms in which volunteers live, eat and sleep, sometimes for days at a time. 'By bringing people in and experimentally overfeeding them, we can make very detailed measurements of the changes in their metabolism as they're exposed to the excess of food,' Jebb explains. In this environment, the scientists can test the roles of appetite regulation, metabolism and hormones.

'One of the things we've already discovered is that our bodies are very badly designed to contend with the high-fat content and high-energy density of the modern diet. It is remarkable how easy it is for us to manipulate foods and to completely mislead the body's ability to detect how much energy is taken in,' explains Prentice. 'If we secretly increase the fat content of foods, we can have an enormous effect on the amount of fat people lay down in a very short period of time. And what's remarkable about this is that the body seems to be very poorly designed to recognize that it's getting fat. It doesn't seem to fight back; it goes on getting fatter and fatter.' However, Jebb points out, some people do seem better able to cut back on their energy intake to compensate once they've put on the weight, while others continue to eat more and gain weight. 'And that might imply that there's some underlying predisposition to gain weight.'

Jebb believes one problem could be that people tend to both underestimate what they eat and overestimate how much physical activity they do. 'What the data seems to show is that as people become heavier, the extent to which they underestimate their food intake does appear to increase. And this can be for a whole variety of reasons,' she says. 'I think it's natural that we all tend to remember the days when we were good and stuck to our weight control plan, if you like. But what we forget are the days when we ate more than that. And so people might perceive that in general they're doing all the right things, but forget the times they actually overate.'

In addition, Jebb says, the difficulty is that fat in food is so tempting. 'Fat adds taste and texture to food, and that enhances the palatability of foods. We like the taste of fat.' And according to Professor Philip James, there may be even more deeply rooted reasons that we like fat so much. 'Fat is a very precious commodity in the world that we've emerged from. In the African jungle where people lived on fruit, berries and wild game and where there was almost no fat, the choicest foods were the fatty, flavoursome foods. So I think we actually have brain mechanisms that search for fat, for sugar and for salt as part of primeval survival systems. And now,' he says, 'we're suddenly saddled with the fact that we have a glorious array of different fats and yet we still have those mechanisms burning away.'

Added to this is the fact that the body's appetite control mechanisms just don't seem to recognise when we've eaten fat calories in quite the same way they recognise protein and carbohydrate calories. 'Fat calories can slip into the body almost unregulated and unnoticed,' says Jebb. 'When we expose people to high-fat foods, they very frequently overeat. They consume far more energy than necessary, and we just don't get the same phenomenon when they're exposed to either high carbohydrate or high protein foods.' A feeling of fullness, satiety, seems to kick in after a high protein or carbohydrate meal is eaten, telling us we've met our energy needs. This, she says, does not happen with fat. The foods we are taking in, in other words, deceive our normal appetite control mechanisms.

There is still much work to be done before these complex mechanisms are fully understood. 'What regulates appetite and what makes us feel hungry or makes us feel full is an area of major research at the moment,' Jebb says. She stresses, however, that the amount of energy taken in in the form of food versus the amount of energy used in physical activity is absolutely crucial to the whole issue. 'Body weight depends entirely on the relationship between the energy we consume and the energy we expend. But that makes it sound very simple,' she says. The fact is, she adds, 'there are 101 influences on what we eat and our energy expenditure, and trying to put together the effects of genes, the environment, behaviour, food choices and so on, is extremely complicated.'

Dr Andrew Prentice concludes, 'There's absolutely no doubt that obesity is genetically determined to some extent, and there are many studies to demonstrate that,' says Prentice. 'The difficulty though is the fact that people will use this as an excuse to say, "If it's genetically determined there's nothing I can do about it". And that's not the case.' He feels much more research needs to be carried out into exactly how genes operate. 'There are many ways in which a genetic trait could be passed on. It may be that some people are more or less keen on being active and sporty. It may be that some people have psychological traits that make them binge and become overweight. So, there are many different ways that genetics could lead to obesity.'

There are also, he says, at least as many different reasons why people become overweight as there are shapes of people who are overweight. 'Some are very obvious, such as ladies who own cake shops, or Sumo wrestlers who try very hard to become overweight,' he says. And at the other end of the extreme are rare cases of genetic obesity. 'But in the middle of all that we've got obesities which come from many different causes. Some psychological, some because of lifestyle, some deeply personal which we have great difficulty understanding. But I think by teasing these apart, we're going to make much better progress towards understanding each and every one of them.' In other words, everyone needs to be treated as an individual.

Professor Philip James agrees. 'Some of the super obese people,' he says, 'have a very powerful genetic predisposition, others are overeating as a psychological compensation for all sorts of agonising problems in their own environment and in their past.' Other people, he says, compensate in different ways. 'Some become alcoholics or chain smokers or become obsessive exercisers. I think we have to understand that people need to be considered individually. It's too easy to say, "It's your problem, it's all your fault".'

Big, Bad, Seductive Fat

'Fat is the magic ingredient in cooking. It's what makes things have great texture; it can be a crispy texture you get with fried fish or fried chicken, and it can be a wonderful fudgy texture in a delicious piece of chocolate cake. It also has a way of delivering other flavours to our palate. Think about a baked or boiled potato compared to a wonderful French fried potato; just think about the difference. And the only difference is fat. It changes the texture, it changes the way it feels in our mouths and it just makes a better eating experience,' says Marilyn Harris, a food consultant for Procter & Gamble. 'And,' she adds, 'it's why we enjoy eating all of those foods which we know often are not good for us.'

High-fat foods, it seems, give us that extra buzz. 'So often when fat is used in cooking, or added to food, you get that extra sensory experience. And I think that this makes us feel like we've had a nice treat and we're happy and we're satisfied.' But this is the danger of eating lots of fatty foods, she warns. 'There is a tendency for people to just keep eating them, and of course the calorie content can get to be enormous when we do that. Fat is a very dense form of calories.' Indeed, one gram of fat has nine calories, compared to just four calories each per gram of protein and carbohydrate.

The Non-Fat Fat

Marilyn Harris is one of a team of people at Procter & Gamble who has been working on the development of a calorie-free fat replacement that is said to have all the mouthwatering qualities of normal fat. Called 'olestra', and given the brand name Olean, it is a cooking oil made from soybeans that have been processed and modified so that the finished product passes though the body undigested; the olestra molecule is too large to be broken down by the body's digestive enzymes which break down normal fat, hence how it can pass though the system without having any calorie value. Procter & Gamble has spent 25 years developing and researching olestra, and the US Food and Drug Administration (FDA), the organisation which must approve new foods and drugs as safe before they are allowed onto the market, gave olestra its stamp of approval for use in savoury snacks in 1996. Since then chips (otherwise known as crisps in the UK) and other salty snacks containing olestra have been introduced into test markets around America. By April 1997 over 10 million servings of snacks containing olestra had been sold or sampled in these test markets.

'Olestra is totally unique. It is the first time the industry has come up with a replacement for traditional fat that has no taste trade-off. And the reason is that it's not another sugar or another starch or another manufactured ingredient that tries to imitate the way fat feels in our mouths.' Olestra, Marilyn Harris says, is made from fat; it is a cooking oil. 'It looks like fat, it tastes like fat and comes from fat. When you look at it you know it's oil, but our bodies don't recognize it when it's digested. So it is oil that gives us no fat and no calories.' She understands that people may think it sounds too good to be true. 'I understand that and if I didn't know so much about it and I hadn't eaten so much of it myself, I would share in that.' Harris feels it's wonderful that industry is beginning to come up with ways to help people eat more healthily and consume far less fat. 'But without having to be deprived of the wonderful pleasure of eating good food and enjoying it,' she adds.

Harris travels around the United States giving talks and doing olestra cooking demonstrations. 'Some people call me the Queen of Olean. I've cooked with olestra for 11 years,' she smiles. Although olestra is so far only approved for use in salted snacks and crackers, Harris says it's potential for use in other foods is broad. 'Olestra works to replace the fat in any food, and we've made almost any food you can imagine that has fat in it; we've taken the fat out and put olestra cooking oil in. And', she says, 'the foods taste wonderful.' As part of her cooking demonstrations, for example, she makes fried chicken. 'I can't think of anything better to eat than fried chicken,' she says, but adds that while it's a popular dish, it's also a very indulgent one if you're trying to maintain a healthy diet. 'Especially the traditional kind where you've got the skin and then there's all the fat underneath the skin and then you bread it to make sure it holds onto a lot of fat, and then it's fried in fat. So, you end up with something that's very high in calories and very high in fat.'

But cooking the same dish with olestra, she says, simply takes away that fat content. 'If we start with a boneless chicken breast, completely trimmed so that it's all protein and no fat, then we use the same procedure only using fat-free bread crumbs and egg whites and water,' she explains. Then, fried in olestra, it becomes the ultimate fat-free fried chicken, with, she says, no difference in taste or texture compared to chicken fried normally. 'You get this wonderful aroma that's reminiscent of my grandma's kitchen back home in Mississippi. And it makes you realize what a wonderful innovation this is, that we can duplicate something so high in fat and yet make it so healthy.' For many, this does sound like a miracle, a dream come true. All that delicious food without any of the fat calories.

Dr Greg Allgood is a senior scientist at Procter & Gamble who has been involved in the research and development of olestra for many years. 'It's clear that obesity has reached epidemic proportions, and it's estimated that nearly 1,000 people die each day in the US from diseases associated with obesity; that's one person every two minutes. What we need,' Allgood says, 'are practical ways to help us reduce the fat in our diet. That's one of the most important things we can do for our health. Clearly the nutritional advice provided over the last years is not working because one out of every three Americans is overweight.' Having a salty snack that's low in fat but has the same delicious taste without the calories, is, he says, a step in the right direction.

'The average American eats 25 pounds of salty snacks a year. That includes more than seven pounds of potato chips and five pounds of tortilla chips per person. So having fat-free versions is going to make a real impact for those people who are looking to still eat salty snacks, but cut some of the fat and calories out.' Allgood explains that Procter & Gamble has started by focusing on salted snacks because that's what consumers said they wanted. 'We did lots of surveys where we asked consumers, "If you could have a food that doesn't have any added fat but still has the same taste, what would you pick?" In survey after survey consumers told us they wanted a fat-free potato chip.' He explains that a small vending machine size bag of chips contains about two teaspoons of fat. 'If a person usually eats a small bag of chips every day at lunch, and they switch to the olestra chips, that can have a lot of savings,' he says. Indeed, the estimate is that over the course of a year, changing to the olestra chips would cut out 8 pounds of fat.

Not everybody, however, is enthusiastically hailing the arrival of olestra. Dr Walter Willett, Professor of Epidemiology & Nutrition, and Chairman of Nutrition at the Harvard School of Public Health in Boston believes the marketing of olestra is in fact cause for grave concern. 'This is a product that's entirely new to the human body. We don't handle it; we haven't evolved the mechanisms to process it like we would normal food, and it has really unexpected and dramatic consequences.' The main area for concern, he says, is the absorption of nutrients calls carotenoids, which are antioxidants that help protect the body from certain diseases; studies have shown that olestra may reduce their absorption by the body. Until recently there was also concern that olestra inhibited the absorption of vitamins A, D, E and K, but Procter & Gamble has now overcome this by adding these to Olean; they have not, however, added carotenoids.

'Even the amount of olestra in five or six potato chips a day can reduce the blood level of carotenoids by 20 to 40 per cent. There are dozens of studies that show that people who have low blood levels of carotenoids have substantially increased risks of heart attacks, strokes, prostate cancer, breast cancer and a number of other conditions including cataracts, which can lead to blindness.' In addition, olestra has been reported to have another rather unpleasant side-effect. 'The FDA requires that products containing olestra declare on the package that olestra can increase the frequency of loose stools and abdominal discomfort,' says Willett. 'It's interesting that they don't mention that in any of their advertising.'

Willett is also sceptical about the process olestra went through in order to gain FDA approval. 'Procter & Gamble used every trick in the trade to get their product approved, and of course now is using every trick in the trade to get Americans to eat it on a widespread basis,' he says. 'The fact that olestra was approved by the FDA is indeed very troublesome. In reality, the committee that reviewed this was deeply divided, and individuals on the committee with public health expertise, and training and experience in evaluating risks and benefits for long-term health consequences, were seriously disturbed about the approval and voted strongly against it.'

Willett is also concerned about research undertaken by another major company into a product very like olestra. 'Unilever actually developed a product virtually identical to olestra, called sucrose polyester,' explains Willett. 'Unilever did careful metabolic studies and published the results showing that even small amounts of this olestra-type product dramatically reduced blood carotenoids, and in the last paragraph of their publication they really indicate that they didn't think it was fit for human consumption on a regular basis. And they've not gone ahead and pushed this as a product to be given to the public. On the other hand Procter & Gamble charged right ahead, trying to reduce suggestions that this might be a problem.'

Dr Greg Allgood disagrees, explaining that olestra is in fact the most thoroughly researched new food ingredient in the history of FDA approval. 'There have been more long-term studies than have been conducted before on any new food ingredient.' He explains that these long-term studies have been conducted on animals, but that there have been studies on humans as well. 'In fact millions of people have been eating olestra snacks for about the last two years,' he says, and these tests have measured the effects of olestra on carotenoid levels. 'It's really an insignificant effect. In fact, if you look at the way that cooking and processing of vegetables affects carotenoids, it has a much larger effect than any potential effect of olestra.' In the context of the overall diet, the effect of olestra on carotenoid levels, he says, is going to be insignificant with regard to health. Allgood also suggests that there is no hard evidence that carotenoids are even beneficial for health.

As for digestive effects and loose stools, Allgood says, 'It's very clear from all the research that's been done that there's no increase in digestive effect.' He says the reason there is a warning on the label is because some very extreme studies showed an effect. 'People were required to eat olestra not just in potato chips, but in a variety of foods, and they were required to eat it for 168 consecutive meals. Nobody eats potato chips like that.' In the real world, he says, studies of people eating potato chips showed no such effects. Marilyn Harris adds that she personally has lots of reasons for thinking there has been a terrible overreaction. 'Who's eaten more than I have?' she asks, 'I've certainly never had any problem. So I'm speaking, as opposed to a lot of critics, from experience.' 'It's very clear,' adds Allgood, 'that this is a product that not only has the FDA stated is safe, but that is going to provide real benefit to people by helping them cut some of the fat and calories out of their diet.' In fact, Allgood concludes, at an FDA review of the most recent studies of olestra, which took place in June 1998, a panel of independent experts gave an almost unanimous vote vouching for its safety. 'It was a stronger vote than last time,' he says.

Willett says that, in fact, it is true there's no proof that olestra is harmful. 'Because no one has conducted a randomised trial of tens of thousands of people and followed them for 10 or 20 or 30 years to see whether or not olestra causes or does not cause heart disease, cancer and blindness as we strongly suspect it will. But given all the evidence, the burden of proof should be on Procter & Gamble, not for us to do studies that go on for decades that may well be impossible to do, to prove that it's harmful.' Willett says that, in legal terms, the company is probably quite safe. 'I think they're probably hedging their bets on the fact that it would be very hard to prove that any single case of cancer or heart disease is caused by olestra.' However, Willett says he isn't surprised the company is pushing this product so hard. 'They've invested several hundred million dollars and they want to get their profits back,' he says.

And as for the possibility of loose stools and abdominal discomfort, Willett adds, 'I think that the real problems are for people who don't get those symptoms.' If people experience them enough, he says, the chances are they'll stop using products containing olestra. 'The real danger is for people who don't get those symptoms and go on consuming the product.' Only time will tell, and it will be a while before a product like olestra will be approved for use in the UK.

Low-Fat Foods

While the experts' opinions on issues surrounding weight and obesity differ in many areas, one area they seem to agree on is low-fat foods. Every day it seems more and more low-fat foods jump out at us from supermarket shelves. Whether it's new brands of biscuits, cakes or crisps, or simply revamped, fat-reduced versions of well-known products, all tempt us with the suggestion that by choosing them, we're somehow doing ourselves a favour. Who knows, we might even lose weight into the bargain. But is this really the case? Columbia University's Dr Rudy Leibel believes not. Removing fat from the diet by taking it out of snack foods or adding olestra, he says, is unlikely to have an effect on body weight. 'For the same reason,' he explains, 'that removing sugar from soft drinks and replacing it with aspartame or saccharin has not caused a great reduction in the body weight of the population.' He believes the body 'eats for calories' and isn't easily fooled. 'The body is really designed to feed itself enough calories to support its activities,' he says. 'It isn't fooled into thinking, "I've just had a full meal", even though it had no calories or fewer calories in it.' Hunger will simply return.

Dr Walter Willett believes it is even possible that low-fat products may lead to greater obesity. 'People are given the idea they can eat as much as they want to.' After all, the justification is, it's low in fat. However, he explains, 'Low-fat products may well be very high in sugar and with just as many calories, and in the end if people eat more of them they will get fatter.' When fat is taken out of products often flavour and texture are lost as well, so many are pumped full of sugar to make them palatable. Willett explains that the food industry spends tens of millions of dollars every year doing research to learn how best to exploit our weaknesses and get us to eat more of every product. 'The food industry has probed every human weakness to make foods taste better in ways that subvert our normal defences.' Not surprisingly, he says, 'this rampant explosion of obesity is a consequence.'

He also points out that fat is now seen as bad, the enemy, when this is not necessarily the case. 'The whole idea that fat in the diet is bad really has no scientific justification. We have actually known for decades that there are good fats, fats that reduce blood cholesterol levels and prevent heart attacks, but there are also bad fats, saturated fats and trans-fats.' These are the ones we want to remove from our diets, he says, not the good, unsaturated fats. 'Removing the good fats could actually increase the risk of heart attacks and other serious conditions.' In fact, he believes, low-fat foods and some of the products in which olestra might be used, could actually replace products that contain fats needed to keep us healthy. The new low-fat version, therefore, 'could actually be worse for us than the original full-fat versions,' he warns.

Professor Philip James stresses that energy density, or total calorie value, is the key. Low-fat products, he says, are often enriched with sugar. 'That stacks up the energy density, even though it's low fat. And when you jack up the calorie content with refined carbohydrates like sugar, you get almost the equivalent calories of the fat.' Dr Leibel agrees that low-fat foods are based on the idea that a fat calorie is somehow more fattening than a carbohydrate calorie, and this, he says, it not the case. 'Taken to extremes, there is the idea that you could eat as many pounds of pasta, for example, as you wanted and you would never get fat, whereas if you ate the equivalent number of calories in oil or greasy food you would get fat.' This, he says, is wrong. 'What really counts is total calories.'

Dr Andrew Prentice has carried out studies into how people react when they know they're eating low-fat foods. 'If we put someone on a very low-fat diet but don't tell them that's what we're doing, they will lose fat spontaneously,' he explains. 'What's interesting, though, is that when we tell them what we've done the effect is spoilt. Then they say, "Oh jolly good, they've put me on a low-fat diet so that means I can now indulge myself and go and eat whatever I want to as a treat".' This, of course, cancels out any savings in calories that eating low-fat foods might have made.

'Since the whole low-fat food industry has come in over the past five years, the average weight of Americans has in fact gone up six pounds,' says Dr Catherine Steiner Adaire of the Harvard Eating Disorders Unit. Ironically, she says, this could be the result of a culture obsessed with thinness, and what happens when people restrict their food intake. 'If you don't trust your body's desire to eat a full range of food, and if you begin to restrict or think obsessively about food, you are very likely to binge,' she explains. She believes that the more we worry about what we eat, and deprive ourselves of what we really want, the more likely we are to put on weight. We are, she says, 'irrationally afraid of fat and food.' It's like a backlash effect: we worry, but we end up eating more.

One thing is certain. To date, low-fat foods, low-calorie drinks and non-fat fats have not even put a dent in the obesity crisis. In fact, obesity is increasing more rapidly than ever before. 'But the amount of money that's to be made from producing suitable low-fat foods or items that help one to slim is absolutely incredible,' says Professor Philip James. 'If I wanted to invest in an area cynically, that's exactly where I would put my money, because looking around the world there are hundreds of millions of people who are already obese and we can predict there are going to be another hundred million before too long.'

CHAPTER THREE

FEAR OF FAT

'Thinness has now replaced virginity as the key to a good life. Heads turn and tongues wag and say identical things about the obese woman that they used to say about the sexually active woman. We either idealise people ridiculously because of their body, or we demonise them.'

Dr Catherine Steiner Adaire,
Harvard Eating Disorders Unit, Boston

The *Psychology Today* 1997 Body Image Survey discovered that 66 per cent of women are unhappy with their weight, compared to 48 per cent in 1972. The same study found that 30 per cent of women feel they want to lose weight after looking at pictures of models. In a separate study it was estimated that 80 per cent of 10-year-old girls in the United States have been on a diet. These figures are alarming and show that women and young girls are feeling increasing pressure to lose weight, to be thinner than they are. But where does this pressure come from? What are the factors that are causing females of all ages to be so unhappy with themselves and their bodies? And how does the desire to be thin affect the lives of countless women and young girls?

The Playground Effect

It's Monday morning at a typical state primary school in central London. Fresh-faced children run around excitedly, greeting their friends, laughing, comparing notes about their weekends. This school, like many others in inner city areas, is a melting pot, with children from backgrounds as culturally diverse as India, Jamaica and the north of England. It's like a mini United Nations, except that here ethnic background doesn't appear to be an issue at all. These young children seem simply to accept and like each other for what they are, no questions asked.

Well, almost no questions. There is one personal attribute that many of them agree is an issue, and a negative one: fat. Studies across a variety of backgrounds and cultures have consistently shown that children rate fat as a major turn-off, a disadvantage. One such study, undertaken as far back as the 1960s, asked children to place in order of preference six different line drawings of the same child. In one the child was depicted as physically normal; in the other five the child was given various disadvantages, one being an obvious level of overweight. Results concluded that the drawing of the child with no disability was consistently the most popular, but the most surprising finding was that the overweight child was, by the vast majority, ranked bottom – below drawings of the child in a wheelchair, with a facial disfigurement, with a leg brace and without a hand. Studies have also shown that a figure with a fat shape is often described as 'lazy', 'stupid' and 'ugly'.

In a simulation of an experiment undertaken at America's Yale University, 24 of the London primary school children, aged between five and eight, were shown photographs of four children: a little girl confined to a wheelchair, a little bald boy with leukaemia sitting in a hospital bed, a child from an unusual ethnic background and a picture of a little boy from Manchester called Daniel Hulley, taken when he was four years old. Daniel is considered, by his parents and the medical profession, to be overweight. When asked to choose the three they would like to have as friends, the majority picked the child with the disability, the ill child and the ethnic child, leaving the photograph of Daniel discarded in front of them. When asked why they didn't pick Daniel, the common reply was, 'Because he's fat'.

In the quiet and privacy of an empty classroom, seven-year-old Daniel Hulley is asked to describe what life has been like for him. In

painful detail he recalls, on his first day at school several years before, how his clothes were ripped, how he was repeatedly punched,
kicked and rolled in the mud by his peers. When asked why he
thinks this happened, he replies without hesitation, 'Because I was
fat.' He says quietly, 'I was treated awfully. It made me very angry,
and I didn't like it. People were calling me fat all the time. People
didn't like me.' He describes scene after scene in the playground
and on the street when he was physically and verbally abused. He
describes walking down the street with his parents and time and
again seeing people look at him and hearing them pass comment
about him or whisper to themselves, and all the while knowing it
was because he was fat.

Daniel began gaining weight at the age of two, and reached 8st.
5lb. by the time he was three. His parents were baffled, and took him
to several doctors and dieticians; nothing helped and Daniel was
still 8st. 5lb. by the age of seven. Then they discovered a diet clinic
close to home that had a special programme for overweight children. In seven months Daniel lost 1st., and says the reaction he gets
from people now is completely different. He says simply that people
like you more if you're thinner, that he is far happier at his present
weight and that he no longer feels he's different. 'I'm very proud of
myself now,' he says quietly. But chances are, Daniel will carry the
scars of his torment with him for a long time, as will countless others who have been through, or are going through, similar misery.

The fact is, the students at this primary school, and at Daniel's
school in Manchester, are simply reinforcing what children around
the world feel generally, according to many studies – that fat is a
bad and undesirable thing. And the reality is that, ultimately, children simply reflect the attitudes they pick up from society at large,
no doubt through advertising and the media, through television and
via the adults in their lives. And, whether conscious or not, children
are being given a very dangerous message indeed.

Not only is society encouraging them to dislike and fear those who are perceived to be overweight, it is also clearly giving them the message that to be overweight is bad, is outside the norm, and is to be avoided at all costs. So overweight children suffer bullying, are ostracised and made to feel bad about themselves, and at the same time, *everyone* slowly but surely soaks up the idea that in order to be popular, in order to be successful and to be accepted by their peers, they should be thin. And it is here, for many, that a lifetime of misery and obsession with weight and food and dieting begins.

Yale University's Professor Kelly Brownell has learned a great deal about this by watching his own young daughter develop. 'My daughter Christie, who is nine years old, is at the point in her life when her body brings her many pleasures. She's very athletic and loves to play games and climb trees and run and do things like that. So, at this point, she is friends with her body,' he says. However, even at this young age, Brownell can see that his daughter's easygoing attitude is beginning to change.

'She's now comparing herself to models she sees in magazines and she's comparing herself to Barbie dolls, and doing so unfavourably. If she is a typical young female, the war with her body will begin at puberty, because at that time there will be so much pressure to be thin, and sensitivity about the way one looks becomes very extreme.' Brownell points out that, ironically, this is the time when the body is naturally developing and laying down more fat, and yet it is also when young women begin to feel this enormous pressure to be thin. 'The body and the culture are moving in opposite directions,' he says. 'For many females, puberty begins a fight between the woman and her body that never ends. People deserve to be happy about the way they look, they deserve to feel that their body is their friend rather than their foe, but it just isn't happening, and there is no sign that the pressure is easing. The ideals people are exposed to are simply unrealistic.'

As a result of watching his young daughter compare herself to

Barbie, and find herself wanting, Brownell decided to study the physical proportions of this world famous and hugely popular doll, and see how they compared to reality. He and his team took the measurements of a healthy young female volunteer, then measured a Barbie doll. They then calculated the way in which the volunteer would have to change her body in order to achieve the same proportions as the doll. What they found was remarkable.

'In the case of our female, who was 5 feet, 2 inches tall, weighed 120 pounds and was very fit and trim, we found that she would have to change in profound ways,' he explains. 'She would have to stand 7 feet 2 inches tall, her bust would have to increase by 6 inches, her waist would have to decrease by 5 inches and her neck would have to be a lot longer.' And the pressure to reach these impossible standards is unrelenting. The last time figures were reported on the weights of Miss America contestants in the late 1980s, he points out, the average contestant weighed less than the criteria for anorexia nervosa. 'So, the ideals that people are exposed to, the anorectic models, the waif-like actresses, the Barbie dolls, are so unrealistic as to pose a real danger not only to people's self-esteem, but also to their physical well-being.'

Brownell believes there is a truly schizophrenic approach to weight in our culture. 'On one side you have these unrelenting messages to be thin, unrealistically thin. On the other hand you have so much pressure and so many inducements to eat that people fall victim to that. So you have these opposing forces, both very powerful, which are pulling people in opposite directions,' he says. 'Some people yield to it by eating and becoming overweight, which is a terrible problem. Some people yield to the messages to be thin and develop eating disorders, and that is a terrible problem. And almost everyone in between those two extremes is concerned with their weight, worried about the way they look and unhappy with themselves as a result.'

Brownell believes these enormous pressures lead many people

to place their physical appearance at the heart of their self-concept. 'And the problem is that there's often a big discrepancy in most people's minds between the way they look and the way they feel they can and should look. That discrepancy batters self-esteem, very often to the point where it pushes out of the way other positive attributes a person might have.'

The Dieting Generation

Both studies and anecdotal evidence point to the fact that these extreme pressures are leading not only women, but increasingly teenagers and even very young children, to diet obsessively in the quest for the elusive body beautiful.

The young women who attend the School of St Mary & St Anne, a progressive girl's boarding and day school tucked away in the picturesque village of Abbots Bromley in Staffordshire, are able to shed some first-hand light on the immense pressures they face in trying to conform to the public ideal. These well-educated, articulate girls are living proof that there is very little chance of escaping peer pressure, or the pressure that seeps in from society at large.

Twelve-year-old Charlotte says, 'At my last school there was a girl who was very fat, and everyone pushed her aside, didn't want to know her, didn't want to play with her in the playground. They just didn't want to be around her because it was bad news.' She explains that it was examples like this, and her own shaky sense of self worth, that led her to start dieting at the tender age of 10.

'I looked around and I was bigger than everyone else,' she explains. 'I know now it was because I was developing before everyone else, but I thought I was totally and utterly different. I didn't realize what was going on, I was getting rounded and everyone else was thin. My best friend was really, really thin. She could still get into children's clothes, while I was in a woman's eight or 10. And this was when I was 10 years old. I just couldn't believe it. I was starting to get too big, and I just couldn't stand it any more,' she says.

'I looked at myself one morning and thought, "I don't want to be like this. I want to look different, I want to look like my friends." I just looked fat, my legs were fat, I was fat, I had a chubby face and I didn't like it,' she explains. So the 10-year-old Charlotte went on a diet. Now she says she has only dieted a few times, and only turns to dieting when she feels she's getting larger than 'normal', 'because you're normal if you're thin.' Two years on from her first diet, Charlotte is at last happy with her body, and even complains that she doesn't like it when her friends enviously tell her she's thin. 'I'm modest. I don't like to say I'm thin,' she says.

There is a lot of talk about weight and dieting among Charlotte and her friends. 'They'll talk about the magazines they've been looking at, and how there are really thin models in them, and how it's so unfair because they are all so big [in comparison]. And I'll say to them, "Look at yourselves, you're not big at all, you're thin". But they just don't believe me.' Fifteen-year-old Emily backs this up. 'We're constantly talking about the way you should look, about the way other girls in the school look. We'll say things like, "Oh, I really want to look like her, she's really thin".' They also discuss the fact, as they see it, that if you're going to get a boyfriend you have to be a certain size: thin. Emily says that in an ideal world men would be attracted to women because of their personality, but feels the reality is that, 'It's based more on what you look like nowadays.'

The story is the same for many of the girls. Fifteen-year-old Gemma, a talented dancer, admits that pressure to look a certain way led her to diet at the age of 13. 'I started to feel self-conscious and was comparing myself to friends in my dance classes, and I thought I looked just huge in all the mirrors. I was not happy with my shape and I wanted to change.' Gemma lost weight on her diet, and admits she enjoyed the attention she got from friends who noticed the difference. 'But then my teachers noticed, and they said they'd start to keep an eye on me and make sure I was eating properly. That's when I thought, "I don't want to do this any more."' Gemma says that it was negative feelings about herself that led her to diet, and that she is now trying to resolve these in other ways. 'I didn't look at my good points, I looked at all the bad points, I focused on them. Now I realize I shouldn't do that. You should focus on your good points and develop them.'

However, although Gemma says she no longer diets, she does admit to missing the odd meal if she feels stressed or depressed. 'If I miss a couple of meals it makes me feel better about myself.' When pushed, she admits to sometimes feeling guilty about eating, worrying that it will make her put on weight. 'Sometimes I think to myself, "You're going to put more weight on, you're going to start looking bigger, and then you might go back to the way you were."' Clearly, that pressure is never far away.

Mako, a 15-year-old student from Japan, seems to feel it doubly. Not only does she want to be thin because she sees it as fashionable and because, 'You can wear all sorts of clothes if you're thinner', but also for cultural reasons. 'I've found that people in Japan are much thinner generally than English people. I think Japanese people diet more than the English,' she explains. 'So, if I'm going back to Japan then I need to lose weight, because my friends there are so much thinner than me. I was thin before, but I'm not any more.' To the casual observer, Mako couldn't fail to appear anything but a slim teenager.

Perhaps the most revealing interview was with nine-year-old Natalie and her 10-year-old friend Daina. Natalie is very slim and long-limbed, and when she gets older will probably be one of those rare people who is not far off the Barbie 'ideal'. However, she was four years old when she was influenced to go on her first diet. 'I saw this modelling programme on television, and all the models were thin, and they had posh clothes on and stuff, and I decided I wanted to be like them. And that day when I went to have lunch I just decided not to like food from then on.' Natalie says the TV programme literally put her off her food, an effect that is still with her today. 'I eat food a bit more now than I used to. When I first came to this school I still didn't like food much, but now I'm eating more.' She says she sometimes has a hard time finding clothes that fit her because she's too thin, and admits she may have overdone the dieting. 'But', she states, 'I like it. I just like being thin.'

Daina listens while her friend Natalie speaks, but is quick to disagree with her. 'I don't think it's right to go too thin. I think models have ruined themselves because they're too thin. You can see their bones and everything. It's horrible.' Daina has a rounded shape, much more reflective of the size of the average British woman than her friend Natalie. And she says she's happy with herself. 'I am, because that's the way I'm made.' But pressed on this she admits, 'I'd like to lose a little bit of weight, but not too much so that I'm like Natalie, because then I'd think I'm too skinny. There's a nice size that I like, between chubby and thin, but not too chubby really. That's the size I'd like to be, but if I can't it doesn't really matter to me.'

However, Daina does admit to feeling some frustration and pressure. 'It didn't really bother me until about the age of nine,' she says. 'Then one day I saw all these people going into shops and buying clothes, thin people, and I just thought, "Oh, they're so lucky, they can buy everything". I went to try clothes on and they looked awful on me. It really upsets me that they can buy those clothes and I can't buy much because there's not many things for chubby people like me.' And it annoys her when her slim friends, nine- and 10-year-olds, talk about needing to lose weight. 'They always say, "I'm too fat, I want to go on a diet and I want to get rid of this," when they don't need to because they're skinny enough as it is. To me, it doesn't really matter what's on the outside. I think it's personality that really counts.'

Daina, it seems, has managed to sift through the multitude of mixed messages and still emerge relatively happy with the way she is. However, many of the young women at the School of St Mary &

St Anne are putting voice to the feelings, fears and obsessions that clearly hound millions and millions of women around the world, not only in Western nations, but increasingly in developing countries as well.

Dr Catherine Steiner Adaire, a psychologist at the Harvard Eating Disorders Centre in Boston, Massachusetts, has been studying this phenomenon for many years. She says the fixation with body weight is showing up in girls of younger and younger ages. 'It's not unusual for five or six-year-old girls to come home from school and say, "Mummy, am I too fat?" or "Mummy, I wish I was skinny". I think what those girls are really saying at that moment is, "Am I okay? Am I loveable?" Probably something happened at school that day that made them feel bad, like being excluded in the playground, or a teacher not picking them for a part in a play or something. So young girls announce their wobbliness in the same way many adult women do: "If only I was five pounds thinner. If only I had a different body type then I would be happier and my successes in everyday life would be greater."'

By the time girls reach the age of eight or nine, they know enough to realise that thinness is equated with success for women in our society, and because there may be many things they can't work out about themselves or their future, their body becomes something they can work on. 'So they start to look at their body as a way of looking at themselves,' Steiner Adaire continues. 'They literally reduce their self-esteem to their body.'

And this, of course, is just the beginning. According to Steiner Adaire, to be female today is to experience a feeling of loathing towards the body. A study in the United States found that every morning, 80 per cent of women in America wake up and automatically have a private conversation with themselves, using what Steiner Adaire calls a 'language of loathing'. 'They'll say things like, "Oh my butt, my thighs. Oh God, if only I hadn't eaten that last night. Well, I'm certainly not going to wear those pants today, I've

got to hide today", or "Today I'm going to be so good because I was
so bad yesterday when I ate dessert at lunchtime."' Inner conversations like this, she says, are the way in which women across the
world greet themselves, in the shower or as they're dressing in front
of the mirror, every day. 'It's not a language of self-acceptance or op-
timism or enthusiasm about the day. It's a language of self-loathing
directed at their body, their shape, their size. And it is regardless of
what they actually weigh, so it has nothing to do with a health-
related need to lose weight. It's all framed by the notion that, "My
body's not perfect, if only I looked a little bit better then I might like
myself more". Most of the men who love the women they live with
would be very upset if they knew how much they suffer.'

Professor Kelly Brownell offers an even more revealing insight
into this destructive behaviour. 'Imagine the following scene,' he
begins. 'A woman is getting dressed to go to a dinner party and her
husband walks in the room, sees her getting ready, and says: "You
should be ashamed of the way you look. You should be embar-
rassed to be seen in public. Why don't you lose weight? You're so
fat, you're disgusting". Now, most people would think of that scene
and become furious with the husband for saying such demeaning
and cruel things to his wife. In fact, that conversation happens all
the time, but not between the husband and wife – between the
woman and herself,' says Brownell. 'It shows how critical people
can become of themselves because of these messages to be thin,
which are unrelenting and unrealistic. People expect that they can
look different, they think if they don't look perfect there's something dramatically wrong with them, and there you have self-blame
and self-condemnation that can strike right at the heart of a person's self-esteem.'

These 'unrelenting and unrealistic messages to be thin' are
clearly having an enormous and negative impact. But just how unrealistic is this 'ideal' that so many seem to compare themselves to?
Dr Steiner Adaire lists the 'ideal' attributes as follows: a woman who

is about 5ft. 10 or 11in. with a weight range of between 110 and 120lb., and very physically fit. 'And recently larger breasts and a very slender, sleek middle area have been added, plus an air of confidence and total self-control.' She adds that secondary sex characteristics, such as breasts, belly and buttocks were all a no-no until very recently, and in fact, judging by models in magazines and on the catwalk, this androgynous, boyish look is still lingering.

These very specific characteristics, she states, are absolutely physically impossible for more than 90 per cent of the population to ever achieve. 'Maybe 10 per cent of the population is genetically predisposed in a healthy, natural way – that is without having to work at it – to be that tall and that slender. But to be that tall and that slender *and* have large breasts actually diminishes the pool even more, because most people who are genetically predisposed to be tall and thin are not genetically predisposed to be large breasted.'

Regardless of these percentages, a constant stream of images of women who fit this genetic minority – rather than the real majority – is fed out into the world via magazines, television, advertising and in countless other ways. And many experts suggest that these images we see on the catwalk and in fashion magazines play a large role in creating bodily dissatisfaction and obsession.

Liposuction

Louisa McCarthy is a pretty 33-year-old with, few would fail to agree, a lovely figure; she weighs 9st. and wears size 8–10. But Louisa isn't happy with herself. 'I hate my thighs. I'm all right everywhere else, but I just cannot lose weight from that area. The tops of my legs have always been just awful,' she says. 'I really don't look at them unless I absolutely can't help it; I don't have any full-length mirrors in the house and I wear clothes that cover up my legs.' Louisa has tried many ways to get rid of her thighs.

'I've tried various diets and exercise routines that are supposed to tone thighs, but nothing really works.' So, Louisa, a beauty therapist from Hertfordshire, has decided to have liposuction; the fat will literally be sucked out of her thighs and upper bottom. 'This is something I've always wanted,' she says.

The operation is to take place at a private hospital in north London, and Louisa is calm when she arrives. She has already had a consultation with Harley Street twin plastic surgeons, Roberto and Maurizio Viel. They have examined her and explained the operation and her mind seems to be at ease; she just wants to get rid of that fat. An hour later, Louisa is anaesthetized and lying naked in the operating room. The Drs Viel, identical twins who together perform everything from liposuction to tummy tucks and penis extensions, are on either side of her. They begin by making small incisions into her thighs and bottom, then pumping in fluid called Klein's solution, a cocktail of local anaesthetic and saline, which loosens up the fat. Then the liposuction begins. The twins work in unison, each on their side pushing their cannulae rapidly in and out of the holes. A mixture of blood and fat is suctioned out and moves quickly through two clear plastic tubes before pouring into small vats. By the end of the operation, which takes about an hour and half, the vats contain 1.5l. of fat, blood and solution.

Louisa is stitched up and home by the end of the day, and the following day takes her dog for a one-hour walk; remarkably, she has hardly any pain. Just six days later she returns to Harley Street to have her bandages and stitches removed, and the doctors are pleased with the results. As for Louisa, she's delighted. Six weeks on she says, 'I'm thrilled to bits. I can really, really see the difference.' She has bought a whole new wardrobe, including some particularly short shorts, and now happily looks at her legs in the mirror. 'This has really changed my life,' she smiles, then admits, 'I've just gone on a diet to get the rest of me looking as good as my thighs.'

On the Catwalk

It is London Fashion Week, February 1998, and the Natural History Museum in South Kensington is abuzz with excitement and activity: the spring/summer collections are about to be shown. For two weeks every six months, the beautiful people of the fashion world – designers, models, the fashion media, movie stars – congregate to watch catwalk shows staged by the cream of Britain's fashion designers. It is from events like this, and similar ones staged in fashion epicentres like New York, Paris and Milan, that the looks and trends which will dominate the coming seasons emanate. Versions of these often weird and wonderful clothes will end up on sale in high streets across the country not long after the shows, though usually more toned-down and user-friendly.

Although Fashion Week is about clothes, in recent years more and more attention has been given to the women who model them. These days, it seems we know almost everything about them, from their names to what they eat for breakfast, to the history of their love lives. The tabloid press and the public can't seem to get enough. In the 1980s and early 1990s, Christie, Naomi, Linda, Kate and Cindy became household names, and each year a new crop of 'girls', as they are called, is introduced. Whether the current look is grunge, glamour or girl-next-door, the right look is crucial, and though the clothes and hair and make-up may change radically from season to season, there is, it seems, one constant. These models, who stare out at us from magazines, television, advertisements and movies, all have one thing in common: they are thin. And, many experts claim, they are getting thinner.

Backstage, models, designers, stylists, hairdressers and make-up artists dash around in a flurry of activity. Most of the models are teenagers or girls in their early 20s. Some have braces on their teeth and are taking time off from school. Some have left school to pursue modelling full-time. All of them are thin, many of them positively bony. They chat happily together, or into their mobile phones, as hairdressers tug at their locks and mascara and eyeliner are applied. Many of them smoke. Bags of crisps are consumed. Many look like any other pretty girl on the street, until they emerge, transformed, onto the catwalk. Cameras flash, music pounds, the atmosphere is sexy and decadent, and the image of the model as one of the most celebrated icons of the 20th century is perpetuated further.

Vogue magazine is widely recognized around the world as a fashion bible, an up-to-date trendsetter with its proverbial finger on the pulse of the fashion industry. Alexandra Shulman has been the editor of British *Vogue* for the past five years, and in that time has been no stranger to the controversy and great swirling debate that surrounds models and the fashion industry. 'It is true to say that over the past 50 years the models you see in fashion magazines have probably become thinner.' However, she says, 'I don't think that *Vogue* alone is responsible for setting the role model for female bodies. I think it's a complicated spider's web, it's very hard to disentangle where it starts and how it evolves. I mean, in the fashion industry you are dealing with fashion editors, photographers, fashion designers, then there's advertising companies, clients and the general public. There is no one person or group that is determining what is popular and what is not. We all work together in creating the images we create, but if it wasn't something the general public wanted to see, they always have the option of rejecting it,' Shulman believes.

'If, as a fashion magazine, if we come up with things that are unpopular, the magazine doesn't sell, just as if fashion designers design clothes that are unpopular, they don't sell. There is a supply and demand element to it all, and I don't think there is a movement which is forcing something onto the general public against their will.' Shulman believes that the women who read fashion magazines are more sophisticated than they are often given credit for. 'I think people buy fashion magazines as a sort of joyful thing, as a way of switching off and I think magazines have been around for such a long time that, in general, the public is very magazine literate. They know how to decode a magazine to some extent. It's meant to be aspirational, an enjoyable fantasy,' she explains. However, she concedes, 'I suspect that there are some women who this isn't true of, and I think age probably has an element to play. The younger women or younger girls are probably more susceptible to what they see in magazines than, say, a 30-year-old woman, who by this time, one would hope, would have a surer sense of self.'

And this is, perhaps, one of the reasons magazines such as *Vogue* often bear the brunt of the blame for eating disorders such as anorexia nervosa. How fair is this? 'Well, not many people have actually said to me that they've looked at my magazine and decided to diet so much that they became anorexic. The people who I've spoken to who do suffer from that problem have far more intelligent and complex explanations for what has happened to them, and the role that looking at magazines had to play in it. I don't think that children who have eating disorders have them because they look at fashion magazines,' she continues, but adds, 'I'm absolutely willing to concede that once they have the eating disorder, it is possible they will find things in the magazine that kind of feed it. But I'm firmly of the conviction that eating disorders come from all sorts of other things in our culture, and things that are very close to home, whether it be problems at school or in the family.'

Remembering back to her own adolescence, Shulman admits that fashion magazines are certainly influential. 'When I was a teenager, I remember looking at images in *Vogue* and feeling they were like the golden 17-year-old I wanted to be. I'm sure there are 15 and 16-year-olds looking at the magazine today, at pictures of Kate Moss or Karen Elson or Stella Tennant or whoever it might be, and saying, "I want to be like them".' However, Shulman believes it's not the body they want but the life. 'We had a debate in the magazine called "Why are models so thin?", and we talked to two young girls who had eating disorders about their reaction, for instance, to *Vogue*.' These girls apparently weren't just influenced by the fact the models were thin, but by how lucky they were not having to worry about their GCSEs and A-levels, and that by being beautiful and successful and in a magazine the models weren't having to succeed or justify their existence in the same way they were, at school and within their families.

Shulman does realize, though, that there are a lot of women out there who are unhappy about their bodies. 'Women have always been deeply dissatisfied with their bodies. I mean, I think that's what the beauty industry has been about for years and years.' She also believes that the search for a scapegoat, a way of explaining this phenomenon, has grown in intensity. 'It's been fascinating to me to see how often *Vogue* and other fashion magazines, though us in particular, have been seen as a kind of beacon of evil that lures unwilling women – young and old – into these thought patterns or behaviours. But if, as people suggest, women really do feel bad about themselves because of external things like advertising or fashion magazines, they would reject them, and they don't,' she states.

Dr Catherine Steiner Adaire, however, believes that when women look at fashion magazines they may unconsciously soak up and internalise messages which are out there in the culture at large – thin is beautiful, for example – and which can lead to self-loathing and self-criticism. She also wonders exactly who fashion magazines are aiming themselves at. 'I know plenty of women who would love to see a far greater range of women modelling clothes, who would really appreciate seeing women in magazines whose bodies look like their bodies,' she says.

However, Professor Janet Polivy, a psychologist at the University of Toronto in Canada, has studied women's responses to the magazines they read and found something quite different. 'There has been an assumption that the fashion industry is forcing women to become anorexic by exposing them to very thin models, and that these models make women miserable and unhappy,' she says. 'So we began a study with the assumption that dieters would feel bad after they looked at magazine images of very thin women. What we found was actually the reverse,' Polivy explains. In her study, both dieters and non-dieters were in fact found to feel better after looking at pictures of slim, attractive women. 'It's as if these pictures fuel a fantasy of what it would be like "if I were thin and I looked like this", rather than a negative comparison of "I'm fatter than that thin model". We have to remember that people do go out and buy these magazines, they're not forced to look at them and they're not forced to watch television shows with thin people in them. They choose to do this, and perhaps they choose to do it because it's a pleasant fantasy to think, "Ooh, I could look like this, I could look good in that dress". It's a sort of daydream.'

However, Polivy has also conducted studies into how women feel about their weight. She brought female subjects into a laboratory to weigh them, but secretly manipulated the scales so that they read 5lb. heavier than the women's actual weight. Many of the subjects were very upset. 'We found they reported lowered self-esteem and they felt worse about themselves,' says Polivy. The study also found that these women later went on to overeat, compared to a group of women who had been shown their actual weight when weighed. 'But it was only chronic dieters who felt this way. Non-dieters were unaffected by the manipulation of the scale, they didn't particularly care if they weighed five pounds more or not. But chronic dieters were very concerned about their weight. When they were told they weighed more it seemed to have all kinds of ramifications for their view of themselves and their moods and their behaviour, because they wound up overeating.'

Clearly many factors influence the way women feel about themselves and their weight. The fact remains, however, that models in fashion magazines weigh, on average, 23 per cent less than the average woman. As Dr Steiner Adaire points out, women who are born with the very tall, very slim shape so in favour for models these days are very much a genetic minority, a tiny, tiny percentage of the population. It would be impossible for most of us to look anything like them, no matter how much we dieted or exercised. While the results of Janet Polivy's study are interesting, the fact remains that many girls and women, when asked, report feeling pressure to look like models such as Kate Moss and Cindy Crawford. Is it possible that the very fact many women don't, or are unable to, reject these images, is what is causing such discontent? And is it possible that some people do go to extremes in an attempt to force their bodies into this unnatural mould, as a result of outside pressures?

EATING DISORDERS

The Eating Disorders Association defines anorexia nervosa as a potentially life-threatening psychological disorder. The main symptom is the relentless pursuit of thinness through self-starvation. Bulimia nervosa is characterised by overeating followed by self-induced vomiting and sometimes purging with laxatives. Anorexia typically starts during adolescence, though an increasing number of young children are being diagnosed. Bulimia normally starts between 18–25 years, and both conditions affect mainly (about 90 per cent) women. It is estimated that one in every 200 girls in the 15–18 age group in Britain suffers from an eating disorder. According to the Eating Disorders Association, approximately one third of sufferers get better without medical help, one third recover as the result of medical treatment and one third remain anorexic or bulimic even after treatment. Anorexia is thought to have the highest rate of mortality for any psychiatric condition; between 10 and 20 per cent die as a result of their illness.

Anorexia

Rhodes Farm Clinic in Mill Hill, on the outskirts of London, is a privately-run centre which treats children with eating disorders, predominantly anorexia. Almost all of the patients are young girls, some as young as eight to 10, and teenagers, although the number of boys suffering from the condition is said to be on the rise with some studies showing they now make up 10 per cent of anorexics. At any one time, Rhodes Farm has about 30 children in treatment. The centre itself used to be a family home and was converted into a dedicated unit, so that it now has several levels of bedrooms, two classrooms, two kitchens, several recreation rooms, therapy rooms and offices, all set in picturesque gardens with a semi-rural view.

Dr Dee Dawson set up Rhodes Farm in 1990 because she realized that anorexia was sharply on the rise and believed a centre devoted to its treatment was needed. Since then, the number of girls and young women suffering from the condition has continued to rise, and Dawson is particularly alarmed by the fact that she is seeing younger and younger patients. 'These girls are seeking perfection, and from a very young age. I had a six-year-old patient who sat here and cried about the fact she would never be a model because she thought she was too fat. She had been reading magazines and looking at the pictures, her mum was always on a diet, and so at the age of six she'd become obsessed. Without a doubt this problem is getting worse,' she states.

And just what is causing this? 'I think we've become a nation of complete health freaks,' Dawson says. 'We're obsessed with healthy eating, with how much bran we have in our diet and how little fat, how much exercise we take. The media has drawn so much attention to it, to what we should and shouldn't do, that people are totally confused by what's a healthy diet and what's a healthy amount of exercise.' The "good food/bad food" message has got completely out of hand, she says. 'Years ago we used to leave children to eat what they wanted to eat; mothers served up spotted dick and custard and meat and two veg, and our children were fit and well and healthy. It might be okay for middle-aged men and women to be thinking a little bit more about what they eat, but for children it's not necessary. I think we're starting children off on a course of dieting and anxiety about food at such an early age, and it's a great shame,' she says. 'They're getting this from their sisters, their mothers and from constant talk that we hear non-stop about how it's naughty to eat cream cakes, how you must go to the gym and how you must jog, and how you mustn't eat fat, you've got to have skimmed milk and you mustn't have chocolate. They hear it all the time.

'Now, Dads jog, mums go to aerobics classes, and all the fashion magazines and the models on the catwalks and every advertisement you see for jeans or perfume or anything else is telling people that perfection is being stick thin, is having your bones sticking out. You see nothing but underweight, unhealthy models, who half the time cannot possibly be having periods at the weights they are. I could pick up *Vogue*, any month, and I could point out anorexic girls who have eaten away at their muscles. They're not just thin, they're ill. And children see these pictures from a very, very early age.'

Dawson spends a lot of time trying to persuade patients that you do not have to be stick thin to be beautiful, but says it's often an up-hill battle. She recalls taking a number of girls to an annual 'health and beauty' expo one year. 'We were in two minds about taking one particular girl, who had only been in the unit for two days and was horrendously thin and very blue, very cold,' she explains. 'She was very keen to go, so in the end we put her under one-to-one supervision with a nurse. Within half an hour of being there, this girl was approached by three model agencies who wanted her to audition for them the next day. That girl had 17 kilos to gain before she would even get her periods back, but she just burst into tears and said to us, "They want me to model now. What am I going to look like if you force me to put the weight back on?"'

Anorexia is a complex psychological and emotional condition that results in sufferers literally starving themselves, sometimes to the point of death. 'I think there are two reasons why children become anorexic. First of all, they have major problems of some sort, usually within the family. They have psychological problems that they're finding it difficult to cope with. They may be feeling insecure or unconfident, and they're looking for something to change that,' Dawson explains. 'Then, they see the media portray perfection as being a size 10, and they hear so much about how good it is to be the right weight and to eat healthily, and they feel that if they could just be perfect they would have more friends, they would be more confident, and everything would be better for them. They feel this is perhaps the one thing they can control and be good at, it's something they can cling onto when they feel that nobody likes them, that they're not popular. They think, "At least if I can become thin I'd have something that people would praise and admire". It's a way of coping with their problems.'

Dawson believes that it is often this desire in sufferers to be perfect that leads them to getting so out of control. 'I believe they're born with a genetic predisposition to be perfect. They're high achieving perfectionists who probably have a tendency to slightly compulsive behaviour, who will want to get straight As at school and will be very anxious if they don't. Nothing second best is good enough for them, and when it comes to dieting, they can diet until death. I think these are girls who see that perfection is within their grasp, because they are often very pretty, often stunning, and they think if only they could have a size eight or 10 body to go with it, they would indeed be perfect.'

And in pursuit of this goal, many anorexics do their bodies irreparable damage. 'Many of the girls who come here are infertile, have osteoporosis, heart damage, liver and kidney damage. Some of them stop growing and stay very short. People who starve

themselves long-term are really very, very damaged by it.' Many of
the girls weigh between 5 and 7st. Recovery and weight gain can alleviate some of these problems, although Dawson says many girls
risk lifetime infertility. 'And osteoporosis, which is an usually an illness that happens to older women, say in their 70s or 80s, is
something you never recover from. All you can do is contain it.'

The treatment programme at Rhodes Farm, says Dawson, is very
conventional. 'We re-feed the children so that they put on a kilo-
gram a week, and the weight gain is absolutely non-negotiable; they
all have to gain that weight. We feed them quite a high-calorie diet,
about 2,500-3,000 calories a day. On top of that they have individual
therapy with a consultant child psychiatrist once, twice or three
times a week. This helps them explore the reasons why they're so
unhappy, and why it is that they feel starvation is the answer to
their problems. Finally, the third thing we do is give them family
therapy, which is the absolute mainstay of treating anorexic children. They almost all have family problems of one sort or another,
and unless we can make some shift in the family, unless we can
change something, we send these children back to face exactly the
same problems that sent them here, and they're bound to relapse.'
Most girls, says Dawson, need long-term therapy. 'They need two or
three years. We really just give them an introduction to it.'

Dawson also does an exercise whereby she sits with patients and
looks through a pile of women's magazines with them. 'We look at
the models and I point out the ones who are clearly anorexic or
starved, i.e., the ones who have actually eaten away at their own
body muscle, who have wasted muscles; they have a very different
shape from the girls who are naturally thin. For example, the tops of
their arms are thinner than the bottom, and the tops of their legs
are concave. Very, very many models in the top fashion magazines
are clearly anorexic. If they're not anorexic they're certainly starving themselves to a level where they're damaging their bodies. I
would think very many of them are not having periods, they're

risking their fertility and they're also developing osteoporosis.'

Some patients will see the light, but about a third will still decide they're fat, and certainly that they're fatter than these models. 'Many of them suffer from what's called a distorted body image,' Dawson explains. 'They aren't able to see that they're terribly thin.' But, she adds, 'We're not asking the girls to get fat. We are happy for them to be five per cent underweight, because that's the lowest weight that's safe, that allows them to menstruate. At that level they can function. Most of them will never be fat. They will never get away completely from the idea that to be thin is to be beautiful and perfect.'

Dawson says disabusing patients of the idea that this is the right way to look, therefore, is very difficult. 'These stick-thin models are highly paid to walk along the catwalk and look like that, and they are obviously role models for our children. I try to explain to the girls that they don't actually judge their friends by the shape of their tummies or the shape of their thighs, but that actually they choose their friends for their personalities. They will all agree with me on that, but often still think for them that it's important they're a size eight.'

She also tries to explain to the girls that genes play a vital role in determining their shape. 'If you look at the shape of a child, and then her mother and grandmother, they are very often the same. Where we deposit our fat is genetically determined. There are people who have big breasts and small hips and people who have fat on their thighs and their bottom and have very small tops, and very often that's something that's carried on through the family. Girls who are pear-shaped with big bottoms very often have mothers with big bottoms, and even when they are anorexic and totally starved, cold and emaciated, they still have a big bottom,' says Dawson. 'I tell the girls that no amount of starvation or waving your legs in the air is going to make them as thin as Julia Roberts' legs, if that's not the way you were born.'

Simply, she says, 'I'd like people to be at ease with the way they are and the way they look, and not constantly be trying to be something they weren't born to be. I would like adults to question why it is that they feel they all have to conform to being a size 10, and for parents to start thinking very carefully before they talk to their children about what's healthy to eat.'

The Rhodes Farm Day

The Rhodes Farm day begins at 8.00 a.m., when all patients must be downstairs for breakfast. On Mondays and Thursdays, however, the children must report for weighing between 7.00 a.m. and 8.00 a.m. to make sure everyone is putting on the required 1kg. a week. Lunch is taken at 1.00 p.m. and dinner at 6.00 p.m., with all meals later at weekends.

Most patients must eat at least 2,500 calories a day, broken up as follows:

Breakfast = 600 cal. cereal and a 200 cal. muffin or croissant
Lunch = 500 cal. main meal and 500 cal. pudding
Tea = 500 cal. main, 150 cal. yoghurt and 50 cal. apple

Patients are allowed three food dislikes, which must be specific dishes. As the Patients' Guide points out 'you cannot put chips, chocolate and cheese!' There are also mid-morning and mid-afternoon snack breaks, when the children take some of their calories in the form of chocolate bars.

School is from 9.00 a.m.–12.00 p.m. and 2.00 p.m.–3.30 p.m., and during free time patients go on activities such as walks, swimming and horse riding, which are based on a reward system, i.e. the more weight you gain, the more exercise you are allowed to do. Parents are able to visit at weekends and phone at specific times during the week. Once a patient begins to get better, he or she may be allowed to leave the unit and have a day out with their family.

Meal Times

Meal and snack times at Rhodes Farm are a painful reminder of just how strained the patients' relationship to food can be. Often there is total silence around the meal tables as the girls and boys focus on what they have to eat. Many nibble, taking small bites, chewing and swallowing as though it were torture, others work their way through their meals in an almost robotic fashion, feeding themselves stoically until, finally, their plates are cleared. There is a rule that everyone must eat in sensible time and not play with their food, and everybody must finish all that is on their plates before they can leave the table.

Sometimes the struggle gets too much, and someone will break down in tears. The others offer comfort – the spirit of solidarity is strong here – and encourage their friend to keep going, to keep eating. They are all aware that the penalty that comes from consistently being unable, or refusing to eat, is tube feeding – literally having thousands of calories pumped into you intravenously. Though it rarely happens at Rhodes Farm, some describe this as their worst nightmare. At least with feeding yourself you have *some* control. Several nurses are present throughout each meal to make sure no one is able to hide food or cleverly throw it away, and nurses have to accompany patients to the toilet for up to two hours after mealtimes, to ensure no one vomits up what they have just eaten.

Rhodes Farm Clinic: Patients' Stories

Ellie, 16

'I can't remember exactly when my anorexia started, but I know I wanted to change the way I looked, because most of the people that I'm around every day are quite skinny; well, I thought they were, and I thought I looked different to them, that I was out of place. There's quite a lot of pressure at school to look the right way, to be the right person, to fit in.

'So, I went out first of all to just lose about half a stone; I didn't want to lose lots. I cut out chocolate and fizzy drinks and things like that and just ate fruit and salad and that sort of thing. Then I went away on holiday, and when I got back people were still saying I was big, so I started to eat less and less and used to vomit afterwards. This made me really scared and I got to a point where I couldn't vomit any more, so I decided to just stop eating. I had to know exactly how much was in my body. So I cut out eating because I didn't feel like I deserved it. Why should I eat nice things, because I thought I was so disgusting? That's how I saw myself.

'I don't like looking at myself, I don't like what I see. It repulses me, and I feel that it repulses other people as well. I think I'm very fat. It's just how I see myself, and how I think other people see me, and just what I am. In my head, I know I'm really starving and that I'm not fat, and sometimes I feel that if I saw someone else my size, I wouldn't think they were fat. But when I look at myself, I don't see someone who's thin.

'I just sort of always want legs like other people, or a flat stomach like everyone else, because it's just so much nicer than your own, and you think that you'll be happy if you can be like that. I don't know if worries like this are the main reason for my anorexia, but it doesn't help that wanting to be smaller is constantly part of life, that it would be so much nicer to, say, fit into the next size down trousers or the little dress that everyone else can wear but you can't.

'I think a lot of the pressure has to do with who you're surrounded by every day, and if most of your friends are thin, you feel that you've got to be like that. But I think it doesn't help when you've got pictures of supermodels and all of them are very skinny.

You don't get a normal weight, healthy supermodel, they're all underweight and thin, and you kind of perceive that as being the right weight to be. And if you're not like that, not the "right" weight, then you feel you have to lose weight.

'I never know how much thinner I have to be to reach the ideal, it's just always thinner than I am. Even when I've lost weight, there's a moment of happiness but then it turns to feeling like it's got to be more, it's not enough yet.

'Being made to eat is not very nice. Nobody enjoys sitting at the table downstairs and eating the food that's put in front of them. You don't get a choice of whether you like it or not, and you can't get away with not eating, or hiding food, because if they catch you hiding food or whatever, then you're made to eat it again and probably more. But to some people it's kind of a relief to have the responsibility taken away. Before it was us deciding whether to eat or not, and now they're telling us that we've got to eat. But I quickly realised that I just have to do it if I want to get out of here.

'I think I'm one of the few people here with anorexia who can just eat and it's not a problem. I mean, I'm not totally happy about it of course, but you learn to accept food here and deal with it. Food was my enemy for quite a long time, but you get used to having it here, so hopefully when you get out of here and go home you can eat normally again. If we could choose, most of us wouldn't have fatty things like butter. Personally I don't like fatty foods at all. But I guess I overdid the healthy foods by far too much.'

Romilly, 15

'I think it was mainly pressure from school, pressure to be popular, and pressure with my GCSEs as well. It was about a year ago that I stopped eating normal food. I had a routine of going to the salad bar at school. I used to eat about six pieces of fruit a day and that would fill me up and stop me eating a chocolate bar or something, and I didn't eat things like white bread or cakes.

'Where normal people have their little indulgences like a piece of cake or a McDonald's, I didn't. I just carried on eating healthy food. It got worse and worse and I carried on and on. If I ate too much one day, like had some bread and butter, I'd cut it out completely the next. I lost about two stone and people started to get really worried about me. My aunt's a counsellor and she wanted me to go and see someone, and I refused because I didn't want anyone to interrupt me. But my family decided it would be wise if I was referred to a clinic.

'I realise I was pretty much a perfectionist. Before I came in here I had a routine where I had to go to bed at a certain time, had to be asleep by a certain time, I had to do a certain amount of homework and have a certain amount on my plate. If not, everything would sort of collapse around me. I didn't think I was fat, as such, but I just got into a routine and it was something to control.

'Being made to eat here is very difficult. You've really just got to get on with it because it makes it worse if you linger over the food; you just get it over with quickly and don't look at it or anything. I really don't like oil or butter or fried foods. I avoided all foods like that, so being made to eat fatty foods here is a bit like torture.

'Getting to my target weight is a terrifying thought, because I've never been anywhere near that weight before. I just don't want to be that weight. I've put on four kilos since being here, and I look in the mirror and think, "Oh my God, I must look different, there's something there that wasn't there before". I haven't got a hollow any more, I've got bloatedness, and if I feel full and bloated now, what am I going to feel like when I get to target?'

Nicky, 14
'I've always thought I was bad, because when I was really little, my dad used to call me fat. Then, when I was about seven I thought I had to lose weight because I wasn't getting very good grades and I felt that people didn't like me, and I couldn't understand why. I

thought maybe it was because I was fat, and I thought if I lost weight I'd be better and more popular. There were thin people at my school who were popular. So I just decided to stop eating. When I looked in the mirror I saw somebody who was fat and ugly and I had to do something about it.

'It took a few months for me to lose most of the weight. And my parents split up, which made it worse. Then I ended up in hospital, a psychiatric unit, and I stayed there for about six months. I can't remember exactly how much weight I lost, but I did go quite low. When I came out of hospital I managed to keep my weight up for about five months and then I lost it again and I had to go to another unit. I was in there for 10 months, and then I was in another unit for three months. Every time I came out I just kept losing the weight again because I was so unhappy. The longest time I've spent at home is 18 months. I just want to go home after this and never go to hospital again.

'I hate eating, but I know it's not my choice until I'm 18. I hate the feeling after I've eaten, I can't deal with it. If I've had to eat a lot I have such a craving to be sick afterwards, and it's really hard because I can't do it when I'm in here. I've refused to eat in the past and I've been tube fed. I don't want to let that happen again because it's such a horrible feeling.

'I hate gaining weight, it's the worst thing in the world for me. But if I don't gain I'll never get out. I'm going to try and keep it up this time, because I'm sick of being in hospitals. But I'm not happy with the way I look at the moment at all. I know I'm fat.'

Bulimia

Rachel (not her real name) is a 21-year-old student from Manchester, and has been bulimic for six years. For the first three years she would binge and purge once or twice a week, but for the past three she has been far more regular and organized, often going through the binge/purge ritual three times a day. To the casual observer she is a slim, pretty young woman.

'I was athletic at school, and I always felt like I had to be thin if I wanted to be attractive and successful. But no matter how much I tried I never felt I measured up, I always felt fat and unattractive compared to the people around me. My mother started putting pressure on me to lose weight, and I tried lots of diets but nothing seemed to work. Then one day I discovered what I thought was a really clever and original way of losing weight but still eating everything I wanted to – vomiting. At first I'd throw up once or twice a week after dinner, and was really happy to discover I was losing weight at last; the more weight I lost, the more obsessive I got. Then three years ago things started to get really out of hand. I started bingeing and throwing up much more regularly, and would also starve myself for periods.

'I now binge at least once a day, and sometimes up to three times a day depending on what I'm doing and who's around me. My bingeing is very organized. I carefully plan what I want to eat then go out and buy it. If my flatmate is home when I get back I'll hide the food and wait until she's out so I can binge in private. Finally, I'll sit down at the kitchen table with the food spread out in front of me and start eating. Normally it will be a concoction of things like crisps, chocolate, convenience foods, sandwiches, pasta, fish and chips, cake and biscuits – whatever I feel like, but always foods I wouldn't consider eating normally, foods that I think are too fattening.

'I don't really feel anything as I eat, just a sort of numbness or oblivion. Usually it takes just 10 or 15 minutes to stuff down thousands and thousands of calories, but as soon as I've finished eating I feel absolutely awful, bloated and full of dread at the thought of now having to go and throw up. I have to psych myself up to go and do it, and I normally manage to within half an hour of the binge – otherwise, I know the food and all those calories start being digested. I often use laxatives as well, which helps get rid of it all. I used to take about 200 a day, but now if I take them it's only about 100. They make me feel incredibly ill and weak, but at least they work.

'If I know I'm going on a night out, I'll starve myself for a couple of days beforehand and take lots of laxatives, so that on the big night I feel thin. If I feel fat I just won't go out. I can't stand the thought of people looking at me and thinking, "Yuk. She's so fat". I used to go out every night, but now I hardly go out at all. I do make myself go to the gym about twice a week though. I used to go every day, until I realized I was getting obsessed with that as well.

'I am constantly influenced by images of thin women in the media, and I compare myself to other women all the time – always coming off as the fat, ugly one. I just don't measure up. I see models in magazines and wish I could be like them, but then I also wish I could just accept myself as I am. The truth is, though, that I do not see an end to my bulimia. I fear I will have to live like this forever, and I cannot stand the thought of that. My bulimia overshadows everything else in my life, it distracts me from everything I do. I have tried to get help, I've tried treatment, but it hasn't worked. I've been on anti-depressants, but they didn't help for long. I don't get much sympathy from doctors and I don't know what else to do, or where else to turn.

'I have felt depressed and cut off for many years. I'm living a horrible, secret life. My flatmate knows about my bulimia, and one of my friends at university knows, but that's about it. Oh, my parents know, but they don't really understand and we tend not to talk about it. They just don't know how they can help me.

'I know that bulimia is a way of controlling my emotions; by bingeing and purging I manage to cut off all feeling for a short amount of time. I can tell from the moment I wake up if it's going to be a bad day, if I'm going to need to binge a lot. Sometimes I even dream about bingeing. It never, ever leaves me. Sometimes I think killing myself could be the only way out.'

Deanne Jade, a clinical psychologist who runs the Surrey-based National Centre for Eating Disorders, has dealt with many hundreds of cases of bulimia. 'Bulimia, like anorexia, is very complex, but the fact is that no eating disorder exists without a diet having taken place first,' she says. 'Most people who become bulimic discover at some point that vomiting can control their weight. For example, a girl may be on a diet and having cravings; she overeats, feels disgusting and then makes a decision to vomit,' Jade explains. Some try to vomit and find it doesn't work, but the ones it does work for often feel they can now truly have their cake and eat it. 'They feel they don't have to worry about getting fat any more.' Although many bulimics tell themselves they'll only vomit sometimes after bingeing, Jade points out that they are often in a dieting frame of mind. 'And so their cravings magnify and they'll soon binge again, sometimes to bursting point, then vomit.'

And so the cycle continues, until, Jade says, it turns into an addictive process. 'It's a procedure. When they feel gross, full and terrible, they find the purging experience to be healing and cleansing. It's instant relief.' And this relief can be both physical and emotional. 'The bulimic woman learns to use bingeing and vomiting as a way of relieving stress.' Stress often triggers bingeing in the first place; the process of bingeing and vomiting can alleviate that stress.

'Many people who come to me have been bulimic for years and years and don't know how to stop. They could be teachers, doctors, headmistresses, lawyers and bankers, often in their 20s, 30s or 40s,' says Jade. And many have kept their bulimia a closed secret for many years before seeking help. 'They want to be rid of the bulimia so that they can go on a diet and lose weight. They feel overweight and dread getting fat and they think what's stopping them from dieting is the bingeing.' Jade says one of the keys to treatment is curbing the urge to vomit, getting women to delay vomiting for longer and longer periods of time until they can finally eat without needing to purge. It's not an easy process, but if they break the vomiting cycle, on most cases the bingeing lessens as well. 'And in 98 per cent of cases,' says Jade, 'bulimics lose weight once they stop the vomiting.'

In a recent American study, a group of college students said they would rather marry a former mental patient, a cocaine-user, embezzler, shop-lifter, nymphomaniac, communist or blind person, than a fat person.

Who Sets the 'Ideal'?

How is it that this fixation with body weight is spreading so insidiously across oceans, continents and cultures? Who or what is responsible for creating this obsession?

Dr Catherine Steiner Adaire believes there are many powers at play here, involving a complex interaction of social, cultural, political and industrial factors. She also suggests that there may indeed be something rather sinister going on. 'It is not at all insignificant that at the very moment in history where women are finally, supposedly, getting equality and asking for equal access and the freedom to throw their weight around in the world, we have an image of beauty for women that's emaciated,' she says. 'There has been a long history of women fasting, but it is only recently that the emaciated body has become a cultural norm.

'What we've ended up with,' Steiner Adaire continues, 'is the most physically impossible definition of beauty in the history of the beauty ideal. It's not a woman's body, and in the late 1990s it's not even a human body.' Not only is there a huge array of diets and pills and potions luring us with false promises, but, 'there are surgical interventions, with breasts being added on; some women and models even have their lower two ribs removed to be able to compete when hip-huggers and halter tops come back in fashion. Even after a model has been photographed, the image is cleaned up.' Steiner Adaire calls this technological surgery. 'Pictures of models are changed using computer technology. A little cleavage might be added, shoulders might be rounded out, facial hair and blemishes removed,' she explains. Airbrushing away wrinkles, blemishes and even fat is common; there have even been reports of advertisers creating pictures using the body parts of different people; one person's legs and another's bust, for example. And all of this after photographers have already used careful make-up and lighting to take their pictures.

'I think that there is a very unconscious, collective backlash against women's equality. It came into our culture in the 1960s, at the same time the women's movement took off and we were being told that we could be anything in life we wanted to be. And this emaciated image we're now subjected to is the exact opposite of what it should be for women who are full of themselves, in the best sense of the word.' In other words, just as women are striving for, and achieving, well-rounded lives, lives that are full and richly textured, they are continually being exposed to an image that is thin, brittle, and achingly hollow.

'It came with Twiggy, an image of beauty for women that is profoundly disrespectful of women's mature bodies. With this body image came a huge form of prejudice. Prejudice arises when people feel that their turf is being threatened; that someone else is asking for a bigger piece of the pie.' Just as women were asking for their share in life, a completely different, and ultimately undermining, way of judging them came into play. 'The reaction is to pass judgement, based on some aspect that people have little control over. The dynamics of prejudice are such that the oppressed eventually take on board the message of the oppressor. They internalize it and turn up the volume in their heads. When I ask girls and young women how they feel about their bodies, they say they hate them.

That's the way prejudice works.'

Psychologist Janet Polivy agrees the issue is a complex one. 'If you ask five different experts why the ideal body image is getting so much thinner I'm afraid you'll get five different answers,' she says. 'There isn't an obvious correct answer for that. There has been some discussion of socio-cultural pressures to de-emphasize sexuality and fertility in women, and instead emphasize competence and self-control, and one way to do that is to iron out the curves and become very slim and non-sexy. We dress for business in clothes, in suits, that don't emphasise curves; we are perhaps trying to alter our bodies so that they no longer reflect our sexuality, so that women can move into the business world and work alongside men without being viewed simply as decorative sexual objects,' she suggests. 'Perhaps women are trying to look more like men, more straight and tubular. In fact they wind up looking more like adolescent boys, so I'm not sure it's such a great advantage.'

Polivy points out that in studies, when asked to choose silhouettes that represent their ideal body shape, women consistently choose silhouettes that are smaller than the ones men select as being their ideal for women. 'Women are aware that men choose larger silhouettes then they do, and yet they still indicate that their ideal is much thinner.' So, perhaps women in some ways are their own tormentors? 'Women are dressing for women, and women are apparently trying to impress other women at least as much as they are trying to attract and impress men.'

Anita Roddick, Founder and Co-Chairman of The Body Shop with her husband Gordon, has a different view. She sees the ultra-thin body image as a strategy used by big business to manipulate women. 'It's so anti-ethical, so anti-women. There's such a hatred of women's flesh in our society. There is such an incredibly successful campaign that's been going on for years, decades, telling women that they should be alienated from their bodies, that their body has to be a shape and form that is not theirs.' The message is, she says, 'their flesh is gross, that it's in need of repair. We're told we have no value after a certain age, that we should shut up, get a face-lift and diet, and the dieting is probably the biggest single message of all. "Get a diet, you look great when you're thinner. My God, you've lost weight!" It's appalling.

'The media, the fashion industry, cinema, constantly shapes us into thinking we're worthless,' she continues. 'We have to ask why there are so many women in this state of negation about their bodies and their own worth, and the answer is simple: business.' The diet, cosmetic and pharmaceutical industries are huge billion-dollar industries, she points out. 'And the only way you sell a product is to tell women that they are worthless, that they are in need of repair, and that the way to become approved of again is to buy a product. This is simple marketing, a.b.c. If you alienate women from their bodies, or if you control their bodies, you control their minds.'

The Body Shop philosophy is to sell products that are natural, that feel good and that do their job, but it is careful never to make false claims. Roddick says the company could make double the amount of money if it ran advertising campaigns that made wild and attractive promises about its products, as some other companies seem to. '"Buy this product and you will eliminate 40 years of environmental degradation, 30 years of arguing with your old man and kids, plus you will look great and it will get rid of the lines on your face and give you a better sex life," she says, tongue-in-cheek, though the message is clear: we are constantly being sold an image that is impossible to achieve.

There is no doubt in Roddick's mind that this control is deliberate. 'Absobloodylutcly!' she states. However, she believes that if any of these major industries were challenged as to their role in this, they would collectively cry, 'It's not our fault'. 'But the culpability is clearly within the business world, the industries that sell to women, especially in the areas of what they wear, what they eat and what they look like.

'For example,' she says, 'we now have two very successful, fabricated, phoney medical conditions. One is cellulite, which all women have, unless they're skeletal, and the other is ageing, which is a natural process, and yet both are discussed as if they're illnesses and have to be treated, and look, here are the products that treat them.' All of which adds strength and approval to the Western idea that women must live up to a certain image, to certain set standards, in this case to be young and thin. 'We see thousands of ads telling women their flesh is gross and that they should deny their age. To be fat is seen as an illness. If we could deconstruct what the media has done historically, then we could possibly see a pattern to all of this. If we could just tell the people out there who have so much self-loathing, "Hey, it isn't surprising you feel like this when we've had years, even centuries, of constant rejection of women."'

'I blame the media, yes I do. I blame the fashion industry, where to be attractive you have to have no breasts, you have to have no hips, you've got to be so bloody glam. I mean, talk about mad cow disease, it's more like sad cow disease,' she says angrily. 'And I also blame the beauty industry. But I would add another blame onto that, and it's our education. We do not celebrate young women, we don't tell young girls they're remarkable and we don't give them a sense of freedom. We don't help them understand that their self-worth and self-knowledge is all about freedom. Take freedom away and you get inertia, you get despondency, you get despair, you get dependency, the social problems that come with lack of, or low, self-esteem. It seems to be the right strategy to keep women down, an unwritten conspiracy which is about suppressing the role of women. It's about control of women and their bodies. I don't know why they think women are so frightening.'

Roddick admits to being regularly confounded by what she sees going on around her. 'Why is a skeletal body more attractive or more wanted than a voluptuous body? Do men really want to go to bed with skeletons, women without breasts or hips? What is it about this magnitude of flesh that is so gross? What is it?' Perhaps the people who are responsible for shaping our cultural ideals, 'all dropped down from the planet Anti-woman or something and said we all have to look like this,' she jokes, puzzled. 'Why are we not liked for who we are? Why is what we look like so much more important than our wisdom, what we've achieved and what we've said?' she asks. 'We have to take control of ourselves, and our opposition. Women have to start regaining their individual freedom. We have to keep on challenging.'

With the aim of doing just that, Roddick and her colleagues at The Body Shop decided it was time for a revolutionary campaign. They had read an American report about the increase in anorexia and bulimia in very young girls. This report also supported the theory that young girls get depressed when they looked at fashion magazines. 'There is empirical evidence that young girls, when they look magazines and see the models in them, get depressed within nanoseconds,' she states. Roddick and her colleagues held some focus groups of their own, which backed up this American evidence and challenged Janet Polivy's findings. 'Young girls took a look at these fashion models and started to say things like, "What am I doing? Why am I so miserable?" It affected their whole sense of self-worth and self-knowledge,' Roddick explains. 'So we decided to do a campaign about self-esteem aimed at young girls.'

Roddick wanted the new campaign to inject a dollop of humour, and to make fun of, and hopefully shame, the industries that push forward this image of 'coat-hanger models', as she puts it. The team loved the word 'rubenesque' and wanted to create a visual icon that would express it. And so Ruby was born. 'We took an ordinary doll and blew it up, computer generated it, to make it like a Rubenesque statue or painting, lying on a couch and just having fun,' Roddick explains. She wanted this to be about rediscovering freedom, about having a sense of joy and wonderment. 'There should be a sense of humour about life, an engagement of spirit, instead of this suppression of who you are, trying to force yourself to be something you're not.' Roddick sees the thin 'ideal' we are constantly subjected to as being about passivity. 'Everything has to be pale and quiet, without energy. You'll never see an energetic photograph of a woman in a fashion show,' she says. 'And until you can start making fun of their language and deconstructing it, it will go on happening.'

The initial campaign consisted of a poster image of size 16 Ruby naked on her couch, with the words, "There are 3 billion women who don't look like supermodels, and only 8 who do", which was launched in Body Shop stores around the world. 'We launched it in Australia during their Fashion Week in 1997, and the response was astonishing,' says Roddick. The campaign grew from there. A life-size Ruby doll was even taken along to London Fashion Week in 1997 to ruffle the feathers of the fashion media. Ruby has since been launched in over 25 countries around the world, and a second poster campaign has recently been put into action showing a curvaceous, naked Ruby proudly standing up with her arms behind her head, this time adding the slogan, "Know your mind, love your body".

Roddick, like Dr Steiner Adaire, suggests that the Sixties marked a turning point in the attitude towards women. 'During the hippie movement women were celebrating their bodies, exposing their bodies during pop festivals for example. There was love, there was an attempt to live an alternative lifestyle.' Yet at the same time, the media's, and society's, obsession with thin women was gaining momentum. 'What people hadn't worked out then was the role the fashion industry would play. Then, suddenly, there was a clue.' Fashion models like Twiggy and Jean Shrimpton were flavour of the moment. They were elevated to icon status. 'Society started to look up to models as icons, as a form of celebrity,' says Roddick. Today, she says, someone like Twiggy would be shipped off to the nearest anorexia clinic.

One man who was at the forefront of the fashion world in the Sixties is Vidal Sassoon. He now has a worldwide empire of hair salons and products, and, as sponsor of the 1998 London Fashion Week, he is still very much a part of the fashion scene. 'I've known Twiggy for years,' he says. 'She's extraordinarily healthy, with an enormous vitality. No one has ever felt that she was unsexy, not one bit. You do find that models are taller and therefore appear to be a lot thinner,' he adds, 'but ever since I've been working and doing shows, models have always been on the thinner side.' He says that during London Fashion Week he has seen many shows, many frocks and many models. 'I've seen some gorgeous girls,' he says. 'Very few I would consider skinny, never mind anorexic. I would consider them extremely healthy. They have to do about six shows a day, rushing from one show to the next, different clothes, different make-up, different hair. Most of them are extraordinarily healthy and, from my sense of proportion, and the way I look at the aesthetics of it, all rather lovely. At 70 I'm appreciating them even more. They have vital lives and a lot of interest in their lives.'

Upon hearing this description of models and the world they inhabit, Anita Roddick seethes. When asked what she would like to say if she had the chance to respond to Mr Sassoon, she says, 'Up your bum and dream on! He has to spend time behind the scenes, he has to talk to people in the know. The reality is that there is quite simply a huge amount of alcohol and cigarettes, and there's diet pills. That's the reality,' she states. 'My daughter is married to a male model, and his observations of what really goes on are enough to challenge every single word that Mr Sassoon is saying. I think he's living on another planet.'

On the other hand, Sassoon uncategorically rejects the suggestion, embraced by Roddick, that women are judged mainly on their looks, that style and shape has become everything. 'I think that's rubbish,' he says emphatically. 'Now we have women running countries, and doing every conceivable job that a man would do, and in many cases doing it so much better. It seems we're making a case here saying that women are truly ill-treated in so many ways from a physical point of view, from a mental point of view and in terms of their aspirations, when I believe it's the reverse. Of course,' he adds, 'I love aesthetics too, I love to see beauty.'

Despite his belief that the world is women's oyster, Sassoon does concede that many women are dissatisfied with their bodies. 'Everybody wants something else, the grass is always greener and the body is always more beautiful when it's on someone else,' he says. 'Very rarely do you look at yourself in the mirror and say, "Wow! Aren't I terrific".'

Sassoon believes the key to bodily happiness is knowing your body type. 'You have to know your build, your bone structure, and how you look at your best,' he says. 'If the world is getting fatter it's because they're eating too much, it's as simple as that. If you are aware of the structure you belong in and treat it well, you won't get fatter.' He does concede, however, there is a chance that the powerful industry he inhabits may indeed be putting women under pressure. 'I sense that if a young lady feels she has to be bulimic or anorexic to look like the girl on the stage, then we're advertising the wrong model of health, the wrong awareness of self. And maybe something should be done in that area.' But, he stresses again, 'Most of these young ladies, these models, that I meet are quite healthy.'

Sassoon feels that if indeed there is a crisis brewing, with eating disorders on one hand and obesity on the other, education is the answer. 'I still say that if through the schools, as part of the curriculum, we had somebody who really understood what we're talking about in terms of body, mind and awareness of self – if that was part of the curriculum – I think this would eradicate much of what we've been talking about.' In other words, education could help people to understand themselves and their own personal boundaries, and this could help weaken the impact of outside pressures. 'Know your possibilities, go for them, do the correct amount of exercise and eat the right foods,' says Sassoon, adding, 'The mind and body don't always work in the same direction. The mind may wish to get thinner while the body's sitting there getting fatter. You've got to *do* something about it.' And every individual has an ideal shape for them? 'And has a responsibility towards that shape, if they want to have a healthy life,' he says.

Dr Catherine Steiner Adaire, however, believes there is undue pressure on women to 'be good', to stay in shape and control their weight by diet and exercise, and that this is a big part of the problem. In fact, women who are seen as being disciplined and self-controlled are revered. 'Prior to the 60s, women were judged as good women, desirable women, if they were still virgins. If you wanted to have a good life it was very important to save yourself for the man you were going to marry. And all the words used then to describe virgins – self-respecting, self-controlled, intelligent, moral, good people – have now been transferred onto women who are slim,' she says. On the other hand, 'Women who are large-bodied are seen as having no self-control, no self-respect, as not being smart, and as having let themselves go: "Oh dear, oh dear, she's got no self-control",' she mimics. 'Thinness has replaced virginity as the key to being a good person.'

CHAPTER FOUR

FIGHTING FAT

'I couldn't sleep at night. I'd be really hungry, with my stomach rumbling, and my mind would be going over all sorts of trivial things, because you can't rest with those tablets, they make you buzz a little bit. So I'd often get up at two in the morning, put the music on and exercise until four or five a.m.'

Linda Cox

The weight loss industry is booming. In the quest to lose weight, Americans are reported to spend between $30-50 billion each year on diet programmes, products, pills and potions; $6 billion of this sum is said to be spent on weight loss products that are fraudulent. In Britain the total amount spent is in excess of £2 billion. Millions of people across the world are on diets to lose weight at any one time. In fact, a recent *Psychology Today* survey found that 84 per cent of women and 58 per cent of men report having dieted to lose weight. In addition 47 per cent of women and 29 per cent of men who are average weight view themselves as overweight. Many struggle with their weight for years and try a huge number of different approaches to the problem, real or perceived. Some of these may be helpful, others ineffective, some downright dangerous. But what really works and what doesn't? Are there any guarantees?

'My Battle to Lose Weight'

Linda Cox, a 40-year-old mother of three, has struggled to lose weight all her life.

'When I look in the mirror, I see a short, stumpy person with fat legs, fat bum and terrible hair, and it's all my fault.

'Dieting and worrying about my weight has completely dominated my life from the age of 11, when my body started to change. I went from being a skinny little child into puberty, but I didn't know what was happening to me. I looked around and none of my friends were going through the same thing, so I just thought I was getting fat. I thought I had a weight problem.

'I decided to do something about it. Instead of having school dinners, I secretly started to spend the money on fruit; I'd buy a pound of fruit and sit and eat that. I really thought it would help me get rid of the fat, especially on my thighs. Even at that age I thought they were my worst area. Everybody else seemed to have slimmer legs that I did, but no matter what I did my fat thighs wouldn't go away.

'After a while I got bored of eating fruit all the time. I swapped it for meal replacements, and spent a few years on those. I was always aware of food, always careful about what I ate. When I got to about 16 or 17 I went onto slimming pills. I found a slimming place that didn't ask any questions. Looking back, I realise I wasn't fat then, probably about nine stone, the weight I would love to be now. But I got the slimming tablets and I started taking them and after a while they stopped having an effect, so I went back and got a stronger type, and from there I went through the whole range of different slimming pills.

'The pills stopped me feeling hungry, so I'd eat just a piece of toast or a Mars Bar and that would be it for the whole day, and I went for years and years like that. I suppose there must have been times when I got so hungry that I ate too much, but I don't really remember those times. Sometimes my weight would go down, then it would start to creep up a bit, but each time I put it back on I'd be just that one or two pounds heavier than I'd been before. So, as well as taking the pills and starving myself, I started exercising all the time, from the morning on and off right through the day until I collected my children from school. It sounds bad, but I'd exercise and dance in front of a mirror and I'd put a leotard on so I could see what bits I really had to work on.

'Often I wouldn't be able to sleep at night. I'd be really hungry, with my stomach rumbling and my mind would be going over all sorts of trivial things, because you can't rest with those tablets, they make you buzz a little bit. So I'd often get up at two in the morning, put the music on and exercise until four or five a.m. I was a single mother at the time, so there was no one to stop me. It got to the stage that when I did actually eat, it would be something ridiculous like half a slice of toast, but I'd feel so terrible about having eaten it that I'd have to run upstairs and stick my fingers down my throat. It was just backwards and forwards with tablets and sticking my fingers down my throat.

'It took over my whole being, really, it was just constant. I couldn't even enter into conversations with people because I was too busy thinking about what I had to do to get rid of my fat legs and fat backside. I remember one night stopping off at a Chinese restaurant with some friends. I kept thinking, "I don't want to eat". Everyone else was deciding what they were going to have, and I was thinking, "I don't want to eat, I mustn't eat". I went to the toilet and stood there panicking; I just wanted to run out, but I couldn't. So I went back and ordered an omelette and salad and pushed it around the plate.

'I'd like to say that all of this has been to do with health, but really it's because I would like to look the best I can; deep down it's vanity. That said, when I lose weight I do feel a lot better, more energetic and healthy at the same time. When I was putting on weight I'd get out of breath just walking down the road. I don't like being overweight, it's horrible. Just before I joined Slimming World in September 1997 I felt very, very down. I was at the heaviest I'd ever been, about 13 stone 11 pounds, which is a lot at 5 feet 2 inches. Normally I'd lose weight in the summer and put it back on in winter, and that was a regular pattern, but that particular summer

I couldn't seem to lose what I'd gained; I couldn't seem to get into dieting again.

'It got to the point where I was crying all the time. I would cry whenever I had to go out to pick my daughter up from school. I'd worry about what to wear, because when it's hot you show more of your body. I'd have a dress on and I had these big, fat arms and I didn't want to show them. I'd be upstairs pulling the wardrobe out and trying different things on, and my husband couldn't understand. He'd say, "You're only going round to the school for Christ's sake, who's going to look at you?" But I think people are always looking at me. There are people who knew me when I was slim, and in my head I imagined they were thinking, "Do you remember her when she was slim? Look how fat she's got now".

'For me, there is constant pressure. Every time you turn on the television or look at magazines or catalogues you see models with perfect bodies on every page. They model underwear or swimwear and you don't see anyone with any cellulite or fat bits or anything that is slightly out of proportion. They're all perfectly shaped women, whatever the size. Even if it's a catalogue for over-sized women and there's a size 18 model, she'll still be 6 feet tall and perfectly proportioned. No one ever seems to be 5 feet 2 inches and stumpy with bits of cellulite. I always think that my body doesn't look like theirs. I might buy something from a catalogue that looks great on the models but when I try it on it looks nothing like that on me. It is degrading, and I think it's very hard work for women, because you constantly feel bad.

'I don't feel I can ever relax, even just going out for a meal. I worry about what I'll have to eat, and it would be so nice to just go out and eat what I want and not have to worry. But I've always felt I had to worry, to the extent that if I get asked out anywhere I worry about what I'll wear and what I will look like and what people will be thinking about me. I've got a friend who, when we go out, homes in on all the fat people to make herself feel better, whereas I don't look at fat people. I focus on all the slimmer people with nice figures and think, "I want to look like them".

'The truth is, when I look back at photos of myself, I realize that for a lot of the time, I've never actually had a weight problem. Sometimes I'll look at a photograph and think, "I remember I didn't want to take my shorts off on that beach, because I felt I was fat", but looking at the picture now I realize I actually looked okay. In fact I often think, "I'd like to look just like that now". It's like you have this mental image of yourself and when you look in the mirror, you don't always see yourself for what you are. For me personally, when I look in the mirror I see a fat person, and if 10 people said to me today, "You look brilliant" and one person said, "No, I don't like you in that outfit", or "You look fat in that", I would believe the one person.

'I'd like to get down to about 9 stone, because that sounds like a good, acceptable weight. Once you say you're 10 stone and upwards, it sounds heavy. I can remember picking up a newspaper and there was a story about a page three model who had put on some weight. The caption said she now weighed, "a hefty 11 and a half stone", with emphasis on the hefty. And I thought, "Well, that's my weight now, so I must be hefty".

'Since joining Slimming World I've had a steady weight loss, and I can eat so much on the plan; I can't believe I can eat all this food and still lose weight. I think of all the heartache I've gone through, and all the tears, and it makes me feel like I've wasted the last 10 or 20 years.'

Linda's story echoes the stories of millions of women across the globe who every day engage in the struggle to lose weight. It is not surprising then that the weight loss industry is booming, not only in the West, but now in developing countries like China and Korea. Across the world billions of dollars are spent each year on diet programmes, pills, potions and products galore, including diet drinks, in the battle of the bulge. In the UK there are several different diet groups and clubs, but two companies run neck and neck for the title of largest weight loss organization: Slimming World and Weight Watchers. Both offer what are essentially diet programmes, though neither likes to use the 'd' word.

Slimming World has its 'Healthy Eating Plan' which is divided into a green and a red plan. The green is suitable for vegetarians, though members are encouraged to alternate between the two. No foods are banned, and all come under one of three categories: Free Foods (a list of over 130 food items – from lean chicken to pasta to vegetables – of which you can eat as much as you like every day, no weighing, measuring or worrying about calories); Healthy Extras (foods which provide either extra fibre or calcium – three portions a day are chosen from two lists); and Sins (foods, ranging from cheese to pastry to chocolate, which are given a sin value – members can have a daily treat to the value of five to 15 sins.) All members are given a comprehensive catalogue of foods that classify as sins, along with their 'sin value'. For example, a standard sized Kit Kat has 12 sins, but a chicken korma has between 30 and 40 sins, and such an indulgence would involve saving up several days' worth of sins.

Weight Watchers, with its 1,2,3 Success Plus programme, also demands no weighing or measuring of foods, or counting of calories, and is run on a points system. Each Weight Watchers member is allocated a bank of points to use up each day, depending on their weight loss goal, and once they join up are provided with a Points Guide listing over 8,000 branded foods and ready meals. All foods are given a point value and members can either stick to their point allocation each day, or can save points to carry over to other days should they want to indulge. Extra points are given for exercising.

Both companies run meetings for their members, and claim to each have 6,000 of these meetings countrywide every week, basically offering support and advice to members. Currently Weight Watchers charges a £9.00 registration fee, plus a weekly meeting fee of £3.95. Slimming World charges £6.95 to join and £2.95 a week.

The World of Slimming

Each year, on a Saturday evening towards the end of October, the largest hall at the Birmingham International Centre is booked by Slimming World. It is here, in an atmosphere of glitz and excitement, that the company celebrates the achievements of outstanding Slimming World members who have struggled with, and ultimately won, the battle to lose weight. Over 1,000 people, mainly representatives of the company's network of 3,000 consultants, make the trip to Birmingham. They spend the night cheering the finalists on and marvelling at the difference between the 'before' photographs projected onto huge screens, and the slim men and women standing proudly on the stage before them. Almost everybody in that room has experienced for themselves the pain and frustration of being overweight, and the achievements of these finalists inspire everyone.

The awards categories include Mr & Mrs Slimming World, Man of the Year and Greatest Loser, who this year is a 63-year-old man who has lost an impressive 14st. 7lb. However, without question the main event of the night is the Woman of the Year Award. Of the slimming club's 250,000 members, about 95 per cent are women, and the 12 finalists each year are the slimmers judged by consultants around the country to be those who have achieved the most remarkable losses. These finalists take to the stage in turn to tell the audience their tales of struggle and success. Some have lost half of their previous body weight and have had to persevere for years, others have battled through difficult circumstances. But ultimately, all have won.

This night is a heady, dreamlike climax of sorts for many people, recognition of hard work and perseverance against the odds. But outside this hall, dotted across the length and breadth of the country, are hundreds of thousands of Slimming World members who are still engaged in their own personal battles, and who can only dream about one day stepping up onto that stage. And for most of these people, their local Slimming World class and consultant are their lifeline, their ray of hope. Each week, 6,000 of these classes are held around Britain. The format is the same whether the class is in Edinburgh or Essex, and the emphasis is on providing support and advice, but also helping women to feel buoyed up and part of group, a sort of 'we're all in this together' feeling.

Pat Shepherd's class in Chingford, Essex is a fine example of this. Every Thursday morning from about 9.00 a.m., Pat's ladies start to file into the local church hall. At an average class, Pat will have 50-60 women in attendance; she knows them, and all of their stories, personally. A queue forms as people line up to register and pay their weekly £2.95, and finally be weighed. The scales are diplomatically hidden behind a screen, so that no one but Pat and the weighee can see how far round the needle gets. Most people look pleased with their result and there's even the odd shriek of delight; a few, though, look down glumly at the machine at their feet and wonder where it all went wrong. What was it they did over the previous week to send the needle off into the ascendant?

Once the weighing has finished, everybody takes a seat and gets ready for Image Therapy. Pat, 45, stands at the front of the class, chatting away about her week, asking and fielding questions, encouraging general banter; often the group explodes into laughter. But then it's down to business. One by one, Pat talks personally to the members, asking them whether they're happy with their result for the week. If not, she'll ask what went wrong. Some admit to succumbing to the influence of a chocolate cake, or hitting the bottle on a girls' night out, or even feeling down and simply, honestly, overeating during the week and failing to 'stick to the plan'. Everybody joins in on these discussions, offering advice and empathising, even delivering the odd gentle ribbing. The atmosphere is confessional, and there's the feeling that trust is simply a given. After all, everybody's got the same goal: to lose weight.

Many, however, are happy; some have lost 2 or 3 or 4 pounds and can see their target weight getting closer. At the end of each individual chat, Pat asks the women what their goal is for the following week. Anything is fine by her, as long as each person is working towards their own goal; there is no pressure, just encouragement. 'I'm going for 4 pounds next week,' states one woman confidently. 'Well, don't overdo it,' suggests Pat, slightly sceptical. 'Just do your best.'

Pat herself is no stranger to the problems involved in trying to lose weight. She has lived though her own struggle for the last 30-odd years, and personally, she says, she wishes she'd never, ever started down that road. 'I believe that if you never start dieting, you will never have a weight problem. At the beginning I thought I had a weight problem, but now I realize I didn't. If I hadn't dieted then, I wouldn't have a weight problem now,' she states. Pat feels that a lot of people are unnecessarily worried about their weight. 'I believe that women who think they've got 4 or 5, maybe 7 pounds to lose don't have a weight problem. Obviously women who are a stone or a stone and a half or more overweight may have a problem they want to deal with. But I believe that if you're a size 12 and you're happy, don't even try to lose weight.' A lot of women genuinely look good to others, but just can't see it themselves. 'I play badminton with a lot of very fit, very slim ladies who tell me they always have to watch their weight. And yet I've known some of them for years and have never known them to gain even half a pound,' she says.

However, Pat herself admits to seeing her own body as an enemy, something that has to be battled with. 'Even when people say things to me like, "You look fine, you look after yourself, you always look good" it doesn't matter because that's not what I see. I see this overweight person who's ugly because she's overweight. She doesn't look good in anything, and that's how you feel. I have friends,' she continues, 'who say they don't see me as an overweight person, they just think of me as Pat. But I look in the mirror and see a person who doesn't look good, this blob of a person. It's a psychological problem, it's just part and parcel of the way you feel about yourself, beating yourself up, worrying and being very, very self-conscious wherever you go. If you have to go through a turn-stile you worry about whether it will be too tight, or if you're sitting close to somebody, you worry about taking up too much of the chair, and whether the person thinks you're fat.'

The struggle for Pat, who has been a Slimming World consultant for four years, began at the vulnerable age of 16. She gained a few pounds, perhaps 6 or 7, at the time she met the man who would be-come her husband. 'Clothes were getting tight, so I joined a class to get rid of those few pounds, which I did, plus a few extra.' She left the class, but immediately went back to the way she'd been eating pre-diet. 'I put on 9 or 10 pounds, and that was the beginning of the cycle. So it goes on. You go back to class, or you try something new, and the weight just goes on again, but always more than went on be-fore. I wish I'd never started. This is the slippery slope that you go up and down. A 50-year-old lady was recently telling me that she'd been on a diet all her life, and I pointed out that actually, she'd been *on* and *off* diets all her life.'

Over the years Pat, like so many women, has tried almost every way of losing weight, all to no avail, she says, until she discovered Slimming World. 'I've gone to all sorts of different classes, tried meal replacements, and I've gone to diet doctors who gave me pills and water tablets. I've seen people by the hundreds,' she admits. 'Once, after I went to one of these diet doctors, I lost 12 pounds in one week, which straight away should have told me this was the un-healthiest thing I could have been doing. This doctor had given me a letter to give to my own GP, and when he read it he told me if I con-tinued to take the pills he didn't want me as a patient any more, so I stopped.'

These suspect methods aside, the problem with diets, Pat says, is that they work if you're prepared to stick to them, but sticking to them is a lifetime commitment. You cannot simply go on a diet, lose weight then go back to your old habits. That's when the weight comes back. Pat sees this endless struggle to lose weight and keep it off in almost all of the women who attend her classes. 'Even the women who have reached their target weights are always fighting to stay there, and they get very strung up if they put on just a little amount of weight.'

Worries about weight and dieting are the dominant force in many of these women's lives. 'Weight does totally dominate your life,' Pat says. 'It can seem to be a chore to be watching your weight and what you're eating, and to be thinking about what food you're buying.' It's something that's always with you, she says, but despite the struggle involved, losing that weight can be life-changing, and a joy to behold. 'I watch women when they're losing weight, when they're starting to feel good and look better, and their clothes size is going down,' Pat explains, 'and I can see their whole personality changing. Whether they lose 7 pounds, 1 stone or 4 stone, a totally different person emerges. It's like a different personality is unwrapped as the weight comes off.'

While Pat loves seeing her class members lose weight, she admits that thoughts of her own battle are never far away. 'I still have times where I lose 3 pounds and I'm delighted and we sing songs in class, make up songs about how good we feel. But if I've put on a pound for no reason, if I feel I've stuck to the plan, then I get very, very disappointed. There's a lot of black and white, no in-between. I'm either very high or very low about my weight problem.'

But Pat says her own lows don't discourage her class members. 'I think we learn from each other. They're interested in how I'm doing and I believe I totally understand them because I've experienced everything they're experiencing.' And anyway, she tries very hard not to show it if she's feeling depressed. 'If I feel the blackness coming, I lock myself away.' Not that she encourages others to do the same. 'People show a lot of emotion in class. There have been tears, people running out to the loo when you've hit a nerve,' she explains. That said, Pat's classes are usually full of laughter and banter. 'I believe that if you're warm and happy and encourage people, they respond. People do not need to be scorned if they have a weight problem, they need help and support. I'm helping people to achieve what they want to achieve.' Sometimes, though, she has to point out that she is only helping. 'Sometimes I get ladies who say, "I don't want to let you down" and I say, "You'd never let me down. You're on your own quest here, and I'm just supporting you".'

Pat is very keen to caution people, young people especially, who may be tempted to embark on their first diet. 'We're at a time when 16-year-old girls want to be six or seven stone. They feel overweight if they're eight or eight and a half stone, which is so sad.' Pat's daughter is now 16, the same age Pat was when she embarked on her fateful first diet. 'A lot of her friends are six or seven stone, and it's very fashionable to be seven stone, because models weigh seven stone,' Pat says. 'Now, I don't think my daughter has a weight problem at all, but she went through a stage of feeling she was really overweight.' Pat was alarmed, realizing she could see her younger self in her daughter. 'I told her that if she gets to 18 and still feels she has a weight problem I'll help her. But I also told her, "Just go through your life, eat healthily but don't watch your weight and you'll never have to watch your weight, ever."' In other words, please don't start this obsession, please don't start this yo-yo cycle and then you'll have no worries. And, for now, Pat's daughter has taken her mother's advice.

However, Pat admits vanity was her main motivation too when she was younger, but says that as you get older health issues also come into play. 'I love doing sports and I'm quite physically fit, but the things that I do are affected by my weight. Sometimes my knees play up now, and my back, and I don't think it's just my age, it's my weight as well.'

Pat is open about the fact she's trying to lose four stone. 'I put on three and a half stone when I packed in smoking five years ago, and I was slightly overweight before that. I've lost a stone in the past four months, so I have a long run. I always tell my ladies a pound a week for a year would be about four stone, so I'd love to be four stone lighter by this time next year.' But underneath, Pat is feeling enormous pressure. 'I feel if I don't lose the weight now, I'm never going to lose it. I think this is my last shot because I don't want to be fat and 50, and I don't want to be overweight when my children get married. I'm not blaming my weight on giving up smoking any more, that's gone,' she says. 'Maybe I'm facing up to my responsibilities now, and that's what I have to do. It's important to me to be lighter than I am, and I feel I'm going to do it this time. I feel positive about that,' she says, adding, 'I always say to my ladies that if they get that feeling, they should lock into it and not let it get away. Because if it does, you get back on that slippery slope.'

Margaret Miles Bramwell, Founder and Managing Director of Slimming World, also understands the nature of the slippery slope. 'Diets don't work. Anyone can go on a diet and restrict what they eat, often painfully, for a short period of time and they will lose weight,' she states. 'But if you then go back to the way you used to eat, the way you gained weight in the first place, the weight will simply go back on.' And this, she says, is where the yo-yo pattern both Pat and Linda have described begins. 'If you deprive yourself of food, food itself starts to become an issue and you can get hooked on it. Food and dieting start to mean restriction, starvation, deprivation and misery. You're asking too much of people to commit themselves to this nightmare.' And it is exactly because of these negative connotations, the idea of a horribly restrictive regime, that Slimming World does not call its programme a diet, but instead a 'healthy eating plan', which aims to change people's eating habits for life. 'And that change has to be comfortable, people have to be able to live with the change,' Miles Bramwell says, otherwise chances are it's back on that rollercoaster ride of deprivation and misery.

Miles Bramwell started the company in 1969, after struggling with her own weight from childhood. 'I tried everything, from hypnotism to acupuncture, to both together, to almost anything else you care to mention. I mean, we're all looking for a magic wand,' she smiles. She was unhappy, lacked confidence and was desperate to lose the weight. Then one day she realised that what was needed was a change of approach, from one of criticism and pressure to something altogether more caring, accepting and even enjoyable. 'People need to know that their worth is inside them; it's not about your weight, you don't have to be slim to be nice, to be loved and loving. You can be that at whatever weight you are.' And so began Slimming World.

'We're human beings and we want to enjoy life; we don't want to live in a nightmare scenario where you can't eat this and you can't eat that. I mean, the minute someone tells you you can't have chocolate, the very thing you're going to become obsessed with, from that moment on, is chocolate,' she says. 'Our approach is to enjoy yourself, enjoy life, enjoy food, enjoy eating and stop feeling guilty about the whole thing. The whole plan is about freedom. We try to keep it as unstructured as possible, so there's no, "What can I have/what can't I have" battle.' Some foods though, the 'sins' are probably the ones that lead to trouble in the first place. 'We say still eat them, but you just need to eat less of them, less often.' The programme is put together by nutritionists, and the emphasis is on changing the way people eat and their approach to food for the long-term.

Members choose their own target weight if they wish, although some people prefer to just take things pound by pound or stone by stone and see where they end up. But once they get to wherever it is they're aiming for, surely the problem of maintaining the loss rears its ugly head? 'Sometimes people reach their target weight and they think they don't need us any more, which is great if they don't. But sometimes they leave and find that slowly, slowly, slowly the old eating habits start to creep back in and they build and build until they're back eating the way they used to eat, and the weight goes back on,' Miles Bramwell admits. 'Sometimes they get lulled into a false sense of security because on the plan they didn't have to go hungry, and they couldn't believe how much they were eating, but perhaps they didn't realise how important the classes were for them.' Others like to stay on and continue going to regular meetings to keep them in the right frame of mind, something Slimming World, like Weight Watchers, doesn't charge them for provided they remain within a few pounds of their target weight. Some members have been maintaining their weight this way for years; many become consultants.

One person the Slimming World approach seems to have worked for long-term is Miles Bramwell herself. 'When I personally was in the 20-stone bracket, I was very unhappy,' she admits, 'and I found it very difficult to just live a normal life. I found it difficult to buy nice clothes, I felt ugly, I felt I didn't like myself, so losing seven stone has made such a huge difference to me. I didn't have anything to prove to anybody; I just wanted to be a weight I was happy with, so that I could live life, enjoy myself and feel okay about myself. I've reached that point now.' Slim she isn't, but at ease with herself and her weight she seems to be.

The Class of '93

We've all heard the statistics: "95 per cent of diets fail" is the well-used favourite. In other words, most people who lose weight put it back on again pretty rapidly. So, while Slimming World may offer a sympathetic and balanced approach, the bottom line appears to be that it can offer no guarantees in the long term. Ultimately, it's up to the individual. So, if maintaining weight loss is a lifetime commitment, just how many people really do manage it?

Slimming World keeps no long-term records, but agreed to help in the search for the 12 finalists of the 1993 Woman of the Year

Award. Only seven were traceable; the others had moved and lost touch with Slimming World. These seven had, back in 1993, lost a combined total of 55 and a half stone; in the five intervening years they had gained back 14 stone – only a quarter of the original weight they had lost. The average gain was 2 stone. So, to a degree, it seems, diets can work. But just how much of a struggle had those five years been? Two of the class of '93 shed some light.

Ursula Van Leeuwen-Hill, a 30-year-old from Cambridgeshire, was 14st. 7lb. when she first joined slimming world. She lost 5st. 7lb. in a year, taking her down to a trim 9st. She now weighs 11st., and runs her own Slimming World class. 'It has been a struggle,' she admits. 'If you have a weight problem, no matter how much of a weight problem or how much you lose, you have it for the rest of your life. It's a bit like having hairy legs,' she laughs. 'You can shave your legs, but the hairs grow back unless you maintain them. Maintaining your weight is hard work and it's a permanent struggle, but it's definitely worth it.'

Ursula says losing the weight is not the hard part; trying to keep it off is. 'I had a sort of celebration period after I lost my weight,' she grins, 'and put on about half a stone.' She quickly realised that sustaining her weight loss would be a lifetime's work. 'Then about a year after getting to my target, I got married, went on honeymoon and gained 10 pounds in two weeks. I only had one outfit left in my suitcase that fitted me by the end. It was at that point that I decided to go back to class,' she says. 'I've been a member ever since and have been able to maintain my weight for almost four years now. Having said that, I've been up by a stone and a half recently because I just had my first baby. That was seven weeks ago, and I've since lost the weight by just keeping to the healthy way of eating.'

Alison Shadbolt was 19st. 7lb. at her heaviest, and managed to lose 9st. 5lb. with Slimming World, taking her to 10st. 2lb. She is now 17st. 7lb. 'I managed to maintain my weight for about three years,' she explains, 'but then it started to slowly go back on. First a couple of stone, and then I maintained that for about 12 months, but over the past two years it's just steadily gone back on. It was mainly due to overeating,' she admits, though adds that she's also had medical problems which may have contributed.

Like Ursula, losing the weight wasn't difficult. 'I was on a high for 18 months, from the moment I joined Slimming World to the moment I reached target weight. I didn't have a problem losing one ounce of the weight,' she says. 'You get so much support and backing from all the girls in the class. They're all behind you.' But as soon as that support stops, things can get difficult. 'When you stop going you can get really disheartened. I went back to class for a while at the beginning, but none of the girls I knew were there any more, and even though you're still at class you feel on your own again. So I decided to just stick to the plan on my own at home. But it's not just sticking to the plan, it's going to the classes that helps.' And so the weight went back on.

Alison has recently gone back to Slimming World, and says she's willing to spend the rest of her life committed to losing, then maintaining, her weight. 'I've got to,' she says, 'because if I don't I'm going to end up 20 stone again and as miserable as I was before.'

The Guru

Everyone in the United States has heard of Richard Simmons. For the past 25 years he has been waging a war, a crusade from one coast of America to the other. He has produced countless books and videos, appeared on thousands of television and radio shows, and travelled the length and breadth of his country to spread the message that burns so furiously within him. Richard Simmons is the fat people's saviour. 'Three hundred thousand Americans die every year from something related to their weight,' he says. 'That's three hundred thousand deaths a year I want to stop.'

While Simmons' mission is deadly serious to him, his style is legendary. Dressed in the skimpiest shorts and sequinned T-shirts, with trademark big, curly hair, he drives along aerobics sessions at his Beverly Hills gym *Slimmons* with his own brand of self-deprecating, camp humour. He sings, screams, weeps, shouts, hugs and kisses, and the classes love it. Here, there is no emphasis on the body beautiful, no weighing machines, no set targets; most participants are 200lb. and upward. The philosophy here is: 'do the best you can. Everything helps'.

Simmons says he was born into the world of fat. He was 200lb. by the time he was about 14. 'I'd never known anything but being fat, being laughed at. At school my self-esteem was constantly knocked down, but at home my parents never judged me by my weight. They said it was baby fat, but when you go from 200, to 250, then almost hit 300 pounds, it's not baby fat any more.' It was with a rude jolt that Simmons first learned how his condition was defined by the world at large. 'I went to the doctor and he wrote the word 'obese' on my folder, and I had no idea what it meant, I was a kid. I went and looked it up in the dictionary, and saw the most horrifying thing.' Obese was defined as, 'Like an elephant, huge, massive'.

One of the first things Simmons did was develop a coping strategy. 'Every day at 3 o'clock when the school bell rang, this guy called Moose used to come up and hit me on the back of the head with a baseball bat, and I'd be strong when I got home because I didn't want to upset my parents. Then one day I told a joke, and Moose put his bat down. I knew then that humour was always going to be my sword, my shield against cruel people. I became the court jester, and I started to make fat jokes before anyone else could,' he says. He also, however, embarked on years of dieting, laxatives, vomiting and anorexia. 'I went from 268 pounds to 119. I went from a 48-inch waistline to a 26. I was anorexic, I was taking 40 laxatives a day, and when I wasn't taking laxatives I was throwing up. One time I starved and existed on water for two and a half months and ended up in hospital, half dead.'

Simmons decided there had to be another way. Having poked his head into regular gyms before and been too intimidated to go inside, he realized other overweight people probably felt the same. So, 25 years ago he opened his first gym for the overweight. 'The first lady who walked in was a nurse who had been fired from her job because she worked with babies and couldn't fit her hand in the incubator any more. She was 250 pounds and she was my first student.' She told someone else about the class, and without having to advertise, Simmons was on his way.

He spent years doing his own Emmy Award-winning television show, 'The Richard Simmons Show', which gained him notoriety around the world; he has written best-selling low-fat cook books, and produced exercise videos with names like 'Dance Your Pants Off'. He now travels 300 days a year, spreading his message to thousands upon thousands of Americans. 'I cannot believe how many more overweight people are living in this country today than there were 10 years ago. It is shocking to me. When I go from city to city, it's almost as if the same group of people is shipped in. There are so many obese children, teenagers, young adults and older people in America.' He reaches out to people in any way he can, encouraging whole towns to adopt his eating and fitness programmemes. One town that he blitzed recently, 'lost over 3,000 pounds in seven days,' he says. Whether it's talking to crowds in supermarkets or taking aerobics classes in shopping malls, he is determined to get his message across. Twice a year Simmons even takes 370 people on a seven-day cruise with a difference. Cruise to Lose, he says, 'is a cross between a boot camp and Mardi Gras.' It's fun, but underneath the message is clear: we've got to do something about this crisis.

Simmons also spends a great deal of time replying to the thousands of letters and e-mails he receives every day. 'I get about 10,000 letters a month and most of them are sad, crippling, tear-jerking, from all walks of life and all countries. If I do a television show, that might bring in an extra 15,000 letters from viewers.'

When he started his web page, thousands more flowed in. 'And if I do an open auditorium on my web page, the next day I might have 16,000 e-mails. Not little ones just saying "hi", but, "Dear Richard, My husband just left me. I have two children, I'm 300 pounds and I'm on unemployment. I don't want to live. Will you call me?" Some days I make a hundred calls, just pick up the phone cold and dial people. I still call this 600-pound man who I've called every day for four years. I don't give up on people, I'm very persistent. It's my job to convince them that they *can* do this. I have to help these people.'

He points out, however, that many overweight people are up against enormous pressure, often very close to home. 'I'll never forget, I was in a mall and there was a line of people waiting to see me and this lady came up on the stage. She was over 500 pounds and she had to be helped up by a couple of people, and she was crying so much that her eyes just became a couple of slits. I reached out and embraced her and we held each other and she cried and she laughed and we talked for a while. Then a lady came up on stage next and she said to me, "That's my daughter. How could you hug her? She's disgusting". How could a mother talk about her daughter like that? Even in families cruelty is there.' And in the world at large, of course, the problem is rife. 'You see a fat person fall, it's a joke; you see them break a chair or not fit into a chair, it's a joke; you see them eat, it's a joke. Don't judge people by how much they weigh,' he says. 'We look at obese people in America as lepers. I want this abuse to stop.'

Simmons understands that with these sorts of pressures, people can get locked into cycles of pain and despair; they often turn to food for comfort, put on weight and get more depressed as a result. 'It's a culinary catch-22. It goes round and round and round,' But, he says, there are so many valid reasons for it. 'You're in your living room watching television, and you look outside and you see your little girl in the street, and she's riding her bike and there's a truck coming. Your little girl dies and your world ends and your refrigerator opens. Your husband is just driving to work and has a massive coronary on the freeway and dies. You start eating, thinking about all the things you did together. You lose your job and now you're six months out of work. The doorbell rings and it's pizza and fried chicken. This is what happens to people. This is reality,' he says. 'We have to train people at a very early age not to turn to food. Food doesn't have any answers, food is not going to solve problems for you. Food is nourishment, but in America sometimes we use our knife and fork to dig our own grave.'

Simmons laments that of course he is not able to save everyone. 'Last year I buried 40 people I had never met. I had to build coffins two and three times the size of a regular coffin, and buy two or three plots for each. But I gave them their dignity, and that's very important to me. I have seen people up to 1,600 pounds,' he continues. 'They've stopped moving, stopped washing their hair or getting up or driving to work. Once they stop going up and down stairs, their bedroom becomes their whole life and then no matter what you eat, you're not burning the calories and 300 pounds leads to 400 pounds, leads to a wheelchair. The ones I lose, well, they're up in heaven and there's no scale there. But the ones that are down here, I don't give up on them.'

Simmons is well aware of all the paradoxes that exist within the American food industry, and understands why so many people battle with food. 'Unfortunately, we're so swayed. The commercials here are so fabulous and there's so much food, it's so plentiful. In America we're known for the biggest steaks and the biggest baked potatoes and the biggest pieces of cheesecake.' Gaining weight, he says, is big business. 'The food industry is very powerful, and this same industry that gets us fat has also designed food to get us slim, and that is so funny to me. First, they get us really fat, then the same company makes these little Ken and Barbie dinners that your dog would turn his nose up at.' And these mixed messages bombard us from every angle. 'It's "Go ahead and eat", then "Oh my God, you're obese, look at you! How did you get that way?"' It's enormously destructive, but, 'It's sales, it's marketing and it's seductive. You see people on television who are the perfect weight, or underweight, who are pretty and don't have a pimple, and you go, "Oh! I want to be like that. Is that fried chicken ready yet?" or, "Oh my God! I want to be size six! Can I have some more macaroni and cheese?"'

All of that said, Simmons does not believe there are good foods and bad foods. 'I don't believe a hamburger's bad. I don't believe that French fries or cherry pie are bad. It's just how often you're eating these things. Are you eating them at every meal, are you taking second helpings?' People, he says, eat with their eyes. 'Food can sing to you, it can sing you a lullaby. Restaurants are set up to be so enticing; food is almost like a painting, it's beautiful, it draws you into it. And then we say "Oh, you made a mistake, you must have done something wrong. Didn't we tell you when you had that pizza that you also had to walk 52 miles?"' He suggests that, rather than just listing the ingredients and calories on food packets, there should also be a warning about how much exercise it will take to burn it off. 'Let people know that when they eat that candy bar it's going to take two and a half hours to get it out of their system.'

While Simmons understands all the pressures that are out there, he is brutally honest about why he thinks people gain weight. It's about eating. 'Anyone who tells you that they gained weight because these little Martians came and force-fed them in their kitchen is lying. They picked up the menu and they ordered sauces and desserts and didn't watch what they were eating. People eat when they're happy, when they're sad, when they're bored, and suddenly they become a robot because all they're doing is eating and watching television.' And the reality is, there are no quick fixes. Simmons does not believe that pills and developing products like olestra, the 'non-fat fat', are the answer. 'Why put out all this artificial stuff, all these pills and stuff you can't pronounce? It used to take years of development before a new pill or a product would come out, but not any more.' Now, he says, these products quickly come and go from the marketplace, offering consumers new hope of a quick fix. 'But it's just another ride at the amusement park, just another roller-coaster,' he says. 'It's another diet hotel you stop at to try the next new thing.'

Really, he says, the answer, though it requires effort, is simple. 'Watch your portions, don't eat late at night, do your exercise and like yourself. That's the real secret, and that is something you can't buy; it's something you have to learn.' Education, Simmons believes, is key. He's been doing his bit for 25 years, and believes it's well beyond time that the government got involved too. 'We wait too late to educate people. We have to get them early. Overweight children become overweight adults, and uneducated children become overweight adults,' he says. Teaching people about themselves and their bodies, funding PE in schools and setting higher standards for the food industry would all help. 'Yes, I want man to go to space. Yes, there's global warming. All those things are important.' But what about investing in people? he asks. 'All over the world human beings are suffering because of this.'

With such pressure, discrimination and neglect around us, it's easy to give into the temptation to blame other people for our problems, Simmons says. But, 'the bottom line is that this is you, and you've got to take you and do the very best with it. You may be different, you may not be that perfect piece that fits in the puzzle, but you're you, and you're all you've got,' he says. 'My whole life is dedicated to making people love themselves. We don't love ourselves. Half my life now, for 25 years, I've been begging people to listen to me. You are worth it, you can do this.

'Every phone call I make, every class I teach, every city I go to and every lecture I do is to get people excited about life, excited about their potential and their future. I'm always the optimist,' he continues. 'I sit and cry when I read my letters, and I sit and cry with these people and I hold their hands and I hug them and I do believe there can be a turnaround. When I'm in the middle of a mall and there's 5,000 people, I know that when they get in their cars and they arrange their rear-view mirrors and catch sight of themselves for a second, they look at themselves and say, "Richard's right. I'm not a bad person. Those people who told me I was bad and stupid and ugly, they were wrong. I am somebody and I'm going to make myself better".'

The Weigh Down Workshop

While Richard Simmons spreads his message across the vast land that is the United States, another message, another approach to weight loss, is growing in strength daily. It's called The Weigh Down Workshop Inc. and the question at the centre of its philosophy is, 'Isn't your desire to overeat really spiritual hunger?'

Gwen Shamblin, a registered dietician who specializes in weight control, founded The Weigh Down Workshop back in 1986 following her own personal struggle with her weight. Like so many others before her, she had tried just about every way of losing weight, but nothing provided lasting success. 'I was a dietician, I was overweight, and I knew no end of fullness. I could sit down and eat large volumes of food,' she says. So one day she decided to watch a skinny friend eat, to try and work out what this woman was doing differently. 'We went to a local hamburger store and she had eaten only half of her burger by the time I'd consumed all of mine, plus my fries and my milkshake. I was nursing a diet drink when my friend did something really strange. She started to wrap the rest of her burger up to throw it away. I said, "What's in your mind? What's in your heart? Why are you able to throw this food away?"' Shamblin admits she really wanted to eat the rest of that burger and that she could easily have finished off any of the food left by her fellow diners. But her friend answered simply, 'I do not want it.'

'I thought that the answer, then, was to just cut the amount of food I was eating in half,' Shamblin remembers. 'I tried that, and I lost weight and I realised that I was simply eating within the parameters of hunger and fullness.' She tried this approach on other people but found that a lot of the time they would simply gain back any weight they had lost. 'I realized the problem lay even deeper than that. Firstly, our parents have taught us to bow down to food. "You'd better clean your plate, you'd better not waste your food". This is saying that the food is more important than the individual. Fact number two is that once we start bowing down to food, and it accumulates on our hips and our guts, we get desperate.' And it is that desperation that leads millions of Americans to the weight loss centres that pop up on every corner. 'Dieting is something that makes you fall more in love with food, and yet it's asking you not to eat it. Dieting teaches us to focus on food. We're looking at pictures of what we should eat, what we shouldn't eat. So by 10 o'clock at night, people cannot stop. They start eating at 5 o'clock when they get home and they eat until they fall asleep. And they don't know why.

'When the pan of brownies calls our name, we say, "Yes, pan of brownies" and when the number three combo calls our name when we're driving down the street, we say, "Yes, number three combo".' Shamblin says the bottom line is that people need to shift their focus away from food. 'Food robs people of their self-esteem, it's a parasitic leech that robs them of their happiness, distorts their looks, and even puts a wedge between them and their spouse a lot of the time. Food robs them blind.'

As a little girl Shamblin had always been in love with God, and discovered that her own focus on God was beginning to help her in her struggle. 'I almost stumbled across this way. I started to help people take the focus off food and focus on God instead. And people were coming back and telling me their whole lives had changed.' There is nothing wrong with food, Shamblin says, after all, God created it. 'He makes everything on the earth, wonderful looking food, wonderful looking this and that. And he puts us down here and allows us to flirt with food, but unfortunately some of us have fallen in love with it, and almost become married to it,' she says. 'And he's saying, "Look, I can do better than that. Come and find out and taste and see that I'm good, and learn that if you open your mouth I will fill it". We are teaching people to love God and enjoy his food. We are putting food back into perspective and helping people to respond to physiological hunger.' And when they do, they eat about one third of what they would normally eat, and lose weight, says Shamblin.

Transferring affections, however, isn't as easy as it sounds. 'This incredible urge to eat, this head hunger, it's a monster and it's strong. It's a wanton feeling; you want more. Some people give over to food, some alcohol, some sexual lust, some power, some money. Anything could fill up this wanton feeling. What we're telling people is, if your stomach is satisfied but you want to continue to eat, turn to God instead. When I first started I would hand people a Bible and say, "Here, go and chew on this", and they might laugh at me, but they would come back weeping because they had found that relationship with God.'

Shamblin spends time explaining to people what they've been doing to themselves all this time, trying to fill up this emotional and spiritual void with food. At first many people say, 'It doesn't seem believable that this cheesedip, this brownie and all this rocky road ice-cream I eat at 10 o'clock at night could be replaced by God'. Shamblin points out that once they've eaten all this stuff, they feel terrible. 'And what's so wonderful is that God can make you feel better than that. I'm not telling people to stop bingeing; I'm saying binge out on God.'

According to Shamblin, the popularity of the Weigh Down programme has grown enormously over the past five years. 'It's now in 15,000 locations in 60 countries, and growing rapidly.' Shamblin estimates that 50-100 new classes start somewhere in the world every day, and says they often receive about 2,000 phone calls a day at the company's headquarters in Franklin, Tennessee. In addition, Shamblin has written a best-selling book that sold approximately 400,000 copies within its first year on the shelves. The Weigh Down Workshop programme itself takes 12 weeks, and costs $103. On joining, people are provided with 12 audio tapes recorded by Shamblin which outline the programme and include scripture readings and facts about food and the human body. A special workbook also covers these things, and provides space for personal journal entries. Then, at each of the weekly meetings, members watch one of 12 videos presented by Shamblin, again outlining various aspects of the programme. As with other programmes, the weekly meetings provide discussion and support; here they also include prayer and scripture readings. If, after 12 weeks people feel they want to go through the course again they can do so at a reduced cost; after that they can return any time they wish for free.

People following the Weigh Down diet are urged to eat whatever they like. 'We're teaching people to go to restaurants and order exactly what they want to eat, and what their body seems to be calling for. And that may be a burrito supreme with extra sour cream or a barbecue or it could be Chinese food.' There's no messy calorie or fat counting; people are free to eat whatever they desire – within the parameters of hunger and fullness. 'They're not just eating lettuce with low-calorie dressing. If they want a salad they're putting real blue cheese dressing on it, and savouring every bite.' And despite eating these kinds of foods, the key to weight loss is that people are eating about a half to a third of the volume they used to eat and with no desire to eat more.

Shamblin reports weight losses of up to 150 and 200lb. 'By being able to transfer a relationship with food to a relationship with God, they're no longer desiring the food,' she says. 'Their bodies are becoming thinner, their cholesterol rates are dropping, their blood sugar levels are returning to normal.' And people are only responding to physical hunger every time they eat.

'I can now stop in the middle of a hamburger, and it's repulsive for me to continue to eat the second half of that hamburger because I'm not loving it any more,' says Shamblin. 'I'm in love with God, and I don't need that hamburger to fill up my heart, and so it's not interesting to me. It would be like if you had a crush on some guy in high school, but one day a new guy walks in and you don't even want the old one to call your name, or write you letters. You're after the new guy, you've forgotten the old.' So God is the new guy? 'Yes, the new guy is God for me. Back when I had this old relationship with food I would get out of bed and put in a good morning's work if I could just get to that food at noon, and then I could finish the afternoon's work if I could just get to the food in the evening. Now, I think about God when I get out of bed. God is my morning, he's my noon, he's my night.'

The Weigh Down Member

In 1994 31-year-old Linda Bessell started the first British Weigh Down Workshop in Essex. There are now several groups around the UK. 'I had reached a weight of 17 stone and was absolutely desperate inside. I was out of control with my eating,' she says. She had tried all sorts of diets, but nothing helped long-term; she'd lose weight but always gain it back. 'I had just signed up for a liquid diet programme that was in the paper. It was going to cost me an awful lot of money and time, because it involved meeting at this woman's house on a daily basis,' Linda explains. 'I came home and I just cried my heart out before the Lord and I said, "Lord, you need to show me whether this is the right thing to do or not", and within seconds the phone rang. It was a friend of mine telling me that a woman who was a member of the Weigh Down Workshop was over from America visiting a mutual friend, and that we could go and meet her. I just knew there and then that this was the right course of action.'

Linda believes she got to 17 stone. because there was a loneliness inside her which led her to comfort eat. 'There was a desperation, a feeling of low self-worth and problems in my personal life.' She was already a Christian, but admits there was still a great part of her missing. 'I was actually using food as comfort, telling myself it would make me feel better. But the cycle is that the more you eat the bigger you get and the worse you feel. I do believe that Satan's plan is to actually keep us turned away from God, and in his way Satan would use the fact that I was finding food a comfort for his own ends,' she says. 'There was this constant, "Go on, it will make you feel better" and, "Why not, you deserve it". Thankfully, being wise to that now I can see where it's coming from and keep it in its place.'

Soon after first hearing about the Weigh Down Workshop, Linda and a few others started the first UK group. 'I just knew that God did have an answer to this weight loss issue so many of us have got. I've slowly but surely learned that God loves us regardless of our shape or size, but that he is also calling us to be obedient, and asking us to turn to him for our comfort and our needs.' Linda believes that the success of the Weigh Down approach is that it stops food being an issue any more. Every other diet she'd tried, she says, simply made her more conscious of food and what she was eating. 'I was actually having to make the food behave by counting the fat grams or weighing food or knowing the calorie content of food. With Weigh Down, all food is good, there isn't such a thing as bad food. At home there's cream, there's butter, there's sweets, there's salad, the whole range of things. I've lost weight by eating anything and everything. All food is permissible, but within the realms of hunger and fullness, and I am being obedient and self-controlled,' she says. 'Now I don't feel guilty after eating cake or chocolate. I'm responsible for my own actions, how I eat and when I eat. Apart from actually needing food for our bodies, food is here for our enjoyment.'

Linda has lost about 5st., close to 70lb. 'There have been a few hiccups along the way,' she admits, 'but I've kept over 54 pounds clearly off. I would say most days now, 98 per cent of the time I will be turning to Christ and not to food. There are days when my own will and my stubbornness get in the way, but generally speaking weight is coming off on a daily basis. I still have a little more weight to go, but I know that I'll get there in due course. To solve my weight problem I've realized that I need to turn to God. He is all I need. I don't need food unless it's to run my body as he designed.'

Linda believes God created us in his image. 'He created our bodies to run perfectly and he's designed a system within us that enables us to know when we need food and when we've had sufficient. It's called hunger and fullness.' Linda says God doesn't necessarily wants us to be sylph-like, but that he wants us to be self-controlled, obedient and not greedy. 'So if the end result is that we're walking around in thinner bodies, then I believe that's how God created us. But saying that, God loves us whatever size we are, he just has the way to bring us into a place of freedom, to be free to eat and enjoy the food that he puts before us.'

Linda acknowledges that the Weigh Down Workshop has been dismissed by some as just another American fad. 'Yeah, I've heard a lot of people saying that it's just another American thing, another way of getting money out of people. I can only encourage people and say that it's the word of God, and it really doesn't matter which country it has come from.'

The approaches to dieting examined here are just some of the hundreds and hundreds available at any one time. Over the years thousands of diet programmes, books and products have been tried and tested, some giving far more dubious advice than others; some have endured, others have fallen from favour and rapidly disappeared. In the 1970s and 80s very low-calorie diets like the Scarsdale diet and the Cambridge diet were popular; these were crash diets and involved severely restricted food intake. There have been liquid diets, high-protein diets, high-carbohydrate diets, even a white wine diet and a diet that promised sex could get you slim. Meal replacement diets have always been popular, as has the counting of calories: 'The 800 or 1,000 or 1,500 calorie wonder diet!'

Celebrities have happily jumped on the bandwagon, publishing their own often gruelling regimes and producing exercise videos featuring their slim selves as inspiration. Women's magazines regularly run diets for their readers, and popular daytime television programmes have got in on the act as well. 'Lose weight for summer' is a standard. And the public, it seems, can't get enough. Some of these diets and programmes have been accompanied by promises of dramatic weight loss and over the years, millions of women across the world have been led to believe, to hope, that this one will be different. This time it will work. And some have, for some people. But, according to *The International Journal of Obesity* in 1989, 95 per cent of people who lose weight on a diet do put it back on again; other researchers have put the figure at 98 per cent, while some are altogether more optimistic.

What almost all experts seem to agree on, however, is that actually losing weight, losing fat, is not the most difficult part. Any diet or way of eating that reduces the number of calories consumed to below the level of energy expended will cause weight loss. But, because many diets don't address the lifestyle and eating patterns that caused weight to be gained in the first place, any weight lost tends to be gained back when the diet is finished and normal eating resumed. Maintaining weight loss, it seems, is the crucial issue.

What the Experts Say

Dr Andrew Prentice of the Medical Research Council's Dunn Clinical Nutrition Centre believes one of the problems is that dieting has been over-simplified. 'Diets definitely do work,' he states, 'but I must qualify that. Diets work if you put someone in a metabolic ward and you rigidly control and reduce their calorie intake; people will lose weight, and they will lose it in a perfectly predictable way. However, it's true to say that very often diets don't work at a societal level, and this is mostly because people don't stick to their diets.' He believes the idea that people can diet for a specific period of time to lose weight and in doing so deal with a problem that has built up over perhaps 10 or 20 years, vastly oversimplifies things. 'It's the wrong way to go about it. What we've got to do is to persuade people that it's taken, say, 20 years to become overweight and it may take two years to get rid of it, but then they've got to fight for the rest of their life to keep that weight off.' And the crux is, he says, that people have to 'reverse forever the things that were wrong in their life for those 10 or 20 years if they want to keep the weight off.'

His colleague Dr Susan Jebb agrees. 'If you look at data from clinical trials in which people have been trying to lose weight, it is quite clear that in the long-term many, many people are unsuccessful.' But, she points out, very often the people who take part in these clinical trials are the ones who have tried and failed to lose weight many times. 'They may be a group that has the greatest difficulty in controlling their weight, a group that is perhaps the most resistant to weight loss,' she says. But in the population at large, 'what we must remember is that in any weight control programme approximately five to 15 per cent or even more are extremely successful. I firmly believe that there are many people out there who gain weight, who recognise there's a problem and who deal with it. And deal with it successfully.'

She warns, however, that there is a danger obesity has been turned into a cosmetic issue. 'One of the things we need to do is reclaim obesity as a health issue. There are a great many people who are battling to control their weight or even to lose weight, who quite frankly are at a perfectly healthy body weight,' she says. 'They're trying to lose weight not to improve their health but because of cosmetic reasons or social pressures.' She feels that in this pursuit of often unrealistic slimness, people can lose sight of living happy and healthy lives. 'And whilst the obesity agenda is hijacked by these cosmetic issues, it's very easy to forget that clinical obesity is actually a serious health risk.' Conveying appropriate messages to both these groups, she adds, is extremely difficult. 'It's important we remember that there is a range of healthy body weights, and that we should be striving to be within that range and not, as at present, striving to be at the very bottom of that range the whole time.'

The fact is that although people may strive to be thin, many are well and truly losing the battle. Indeed, the rate of obesity is rising at an alarming rate all over the world. In 1980, six per cent of men and eight per cent of women in England were obese. By 1998 the number of obese people had more than doubled; now 16 per cent of men and 17 per cent of women are obese, and experts say these figures will continue to rise rapidly. It is predicted that obesity will now double every seven years. And, ironically, this increase has taken place over a period of time in which the Western world has never been more conscious of weight, diet, exercise and the body beautiful.

Yale University's Professor Kelly Brownell believes these outside pressures exacerbate the problems. 'It's necessary to strike the correct and most humane balance between encouraging people to lose weight and achieve a healthier weight if they need to, and not pushing them too hard so they become preoccupied and obsessed with their eating and their weight and their bodies,' he says. 'The message we need to impart is to attain the best weight you can, don't worry about the unrealistic beauty ideals, don't worry about some arbitrary numbers in the tables of ideal weights. Instead, try to eat a sensible diet, get enough exercise to be healthy and see where your weight settles, and that's probably a pretty good middle ground.' He suggests that if a person feels they have 50lb. to lose, instead of saying, 'I need to lose 50 pounds to hit my ideal weight', they can say, 'Why don't I lose 10 pounds and see how I feel there? I'll be a lot better off than I am now'. 'Then they can see if they're able to maintain that 10 pound loss, and decide whether to lose more.' The important thing is, he stresses, is that people make reasonable changes in their diet and exercise but without pushing themselves too far.

'The human mind is terribly important in this,' Brownell says. 'Food has tremendous psychological meaning for some people. For some individuals food is comfort, food is a way of escaping from a difficult world. It's a way of escaping from bad relationships, it's a way of blotting out difficult things going on in life. For some people food is their best friend, and for some it's their only friend. So, imagine how difficult it would be for somebody like that to give up their food in order to lose weight,' he says. 'It explains in some measure why weight loss is so difficult for some people and why they relapse even after they've lost weight successfully. In order to counter that, one has to draw upon resources and strength and support from somewhere else.'

Some people get that support from health care professionals or from their families, he says. 'Some people get it from weight loss programmes, some get it in a spiritual way, or may join a group in a church. Wherever it comes from, I think it's good. If somebody enters into a group where they get strength and support from a spiritual source, so be it. If it works for them I celebrate that.' It is by entering these sort of social relationships that real help can be gained, explains Brownell. 'If they persist over the long term that's even better, because it may help guarantee that once the weight is lost, there will be some support to help keep it off.'

So, the experts agree that keeping weight off is at the heart of the matter, although Columbia University's Dr Rudy Leibel has possibly the most pessimistic view. His 'set point' theory, as explained in Chapter One, suggests that once weight is lost, the body automatically fights to get back to where it was, to its 'set point'. 'This is the reason we believe there is such an enormous failure rate in the ability to maintain lowered body weight in the obese.' By losing weight, he says, the body is actually taken into a metabolic state which is abnormal for it. 'The body resists this as if it were a deformation,' Leibel explains. 'The body in fact adjusts its metabolism in such a way as to resist the new lower weight, and actually cause the individual to go back up to the weight they started at.' Leibel believes, then, that it's really only wise to try and lose weight if it's medically necessary. 'If one is quite healthy at their level of body fatness, my advice is to learn to live with it, accept it and not try to take drastic measures to lose weight.'

This view, however, is thought by some experts to be quite extreme. Dr Andrew Prentice, for example, believes things are not as bleak as this. 'The body does fight back and try to defend itself against weight loss,' he agrees, 'and this makes an awful lot of sense in evolutionary terms. We don't want to fade away quickly when we come to a famine.' But, he adds, 'the difficulty is that some people have exaggerated this effect and raised it as a barrier to weight loss, and it certainly is not that.' Prentice's own studies show that while the metabolic rate does slow down after a period of dieting, it then returns to normal after just a few weeks: 'I've done a lot of work in Gambia in West Africa where we've looked at people who go through an annual hungry season, where they lose a lot of weight and then pile it back on during the harvest season. This is a totally natural biological phenomenal. It's fat acting as fat was designed to act.'

'It would be very surprising to me if the penalty for using our fat stores in the way that they were designed, was that it wrecked our metabolism for the rest of our lives. This simply doesn't happen.' It may make losing weight and keeping it off a bit more difficult, but certainly not impossible.

This is good news, and the even better news is that some feel losing weight shouldn't necessarily be the focus. Professor Philip James of Aberdeen's Rowett Research Institute believes that these days, simply preventing further weight gain is a major success. 'We are still obsessed with the idea of losing weight, yet to stop putting weight on is a staggering achievement,' he says. 'Wherever you are once you focus on the fact you've been putting on weight, that's the point at which to stop putting on weight. That's the first big triumph.' And James believes we far too easily blame the individual for gaining weight. The attitude is, "It's your problem, you're at fault". The truth is, he says, the whole of society is no longer geared to allowing people to maintain a reasonable weight. The abundance of food plus our sedentary lifestyle are at the root of the problem.

As far as dieting goes, James believes that it's important not just to think about calories, but about the types of foods being eaten. 'You can change the risk of developing heart disease and high blood pressure associated with obesity quite dramatically simply by carefully choosing the nature of your diet.' By eating a predominantly carbohydrate, coarse grain, cereal-type diet with lots of fruit and vegetables, he says, you can reap these health benefits without losing a single pound in weight. However, he adds, the good news for obese people is that even small amounts of weight loss can make a huge difference.

'Recent data shows that losing a stone, or 5 kilos, certainly 10 kilos, will have a dramatic benefit.' By adding exercise into the equation, even without dramatic weight loss, there is less risk of developing such conditions of heart disease and diabetes. James feels that pressure to reach low target weights, often attached to dieting, is not only misleading but destructive. 'It's a tragedy that we in the medical profession, backed up by streams of articles, have this idea of a goal weight. It's a recipe for generating people who are constantly in agony.' If overweight people can reduce their weight modestly and change their diet and amount of exercise, that's a huge bonus, he says. 'But the first thing is, don't put on any more.'

This is clearly an important message, though the reality is that people will continue to want to diet. But what if dieting, the very process millions of people put their faith in, really is contributing to the problem? Professor Janet Polivy, a psychologist at the University of Toronto, believes dieting really can make you fatter, and for the past 20 years she has carried out research which appears to verify this. 'The more we try to diet and force our bodies to look like some slim ideal that most of us were never meant to resemble, the more we find ourselves overeating whenever we let our guards down, and the more we end up gaining weight.' Polivy explains that when we deprive ourselves of food on a diet, the body immediately fights back to preserve itself by encouraging us to overeat. 'Our bodies don't know that fashion has dictated that thin is in, our bodies think there's a famine out there. We are fighting against our bodies to try and look like the fashionable ideal.

'And when people finish diets,' she continues, 'instead of maintaining the weight loss they often regain more than they originally lost, so wind up getting fatter and fatter with each successive diet they go on. There are certainly some people who would not be as obese as they are if they had never dieted.' Polivy believes, however, in cases of morbid obesity, that there is often a genetic component at work as well. Their bodies, she says, have allowed them to reach that point. 'Most of us couldn't become morbidly obese if we tried.'

Polivy believes it is very important for people who feel they need to lose weight to think about what they really want before embarking on a diet. 'Are you doing it because you think being thin is going to get you all kinds of rewards? If you think that losing weight is going to get you a better job or a better boyfriend or anything else, reconsider and instead learn to accept yourself as you are,' she suggests. 'Go directly after those things you want.' Losing weight, she says, can be just an indirect way of achieving other goals. If you go directly for those goals, rather than through dieting, you have a better chance of success. However, if people want to lose weight for health reasons, she says, they should first be assessed to make sure they really do have a health problem. 'If they do, they can then deal with their weight in a realistic fashion.'

Drastic dieting or any kind of short-term diet is not the way to go about it, she says. Like the other experts, she recommends a moderate approach, a gradual change of lifestyle. 'Increase your exercise and just pay attention to what you eat so that you have a more balanced, nutritious diet and include all your favourite foods, even the fattening ones. Eat fattening foods at the end of a meal in smaller quantities when you're not terribly hungry for them,' Polivy suggests. 'Or incorporate them into the meal along with other foods so that they are part of your normal life. Don't cut things out that you would miss tremendously if you didn't have them.' Polivy's research confirms that dieters are much more likely to overeat than non-dieters, and that dieting actually promotes overeating. 'People do eat more than they would have if they had just allowed themselves to eat the foods they wanted, but learned to eat them in moderation,' she says. 'Learn only to eat when you're hungry, and to stop eating when you're no longer hungry. I think most people would find that if they were able to do that they would eat less, because we tend to eat past the point where we are satisfied – we eat until we are full.'

Polivy is unforgiving of the diet industry. 'The diet industry is definitely not an industry I admire,' she says. 'It's an industry that makes billions based on its failure to produce its desired effect.' Women in particular are exploited, she says. The more that people fail to lose weight, the more they turn back to the diet industry for help, and in the process hand over yet more money. 'People try again and again. Instead of recognizing that it is the diets that are failing, they blame themselves. I blame the diet industry for making people feel like failures and capitalizing on that.' Polivy says we're led to believe that losing weight is easy. 'We're told by the diet industry, "Of course you can change your weight, no problem, very simple. Just do this and you'll be thinner, happier, your life will be wonderful". And so people have this unrealistic expectation that they can change their body shape, and they blame themselves, rather than the diet, when they're unable to do that.'

A growing minority of people feel even more strongly. 'If any one of the thousands of diet programmes and diet products and pills out there worked, they would all go out of business. All weight loss programmes are evil to me. They all make money out of the fact that fat people are oppressed and exploited,' says Marilyn Wann, editor of US magazine *Fat?So!* and member of NAAFA, the US National Association to Advance Fat Acceptance. 'They rely on their products and programmes not working, because they want repeat customers. Diet programmes, for example, often make claims that they have millions of success stories; the truth is that many of these so-called successes are in fact repeat customers, people who have lost the same 10 pounds five times over, but still keep going back. It's not in the interest of these companies to weed out the repeat customers.' Wann's views are considered extreme by many, but, although *Fat?So!* has a circulation of just 2,000, she echoes the voices of a growing number of 'fat acceptance' activists around the world.

Wann, who is in her mid-30s and weighs about 250lb., says incredible things could be done with the estimated $40 billion Americans spend each year on diet programmes, pills and products – money she sees as completely wasted. '$40 billion would put 800,000 people through four years of college. That's the entire graduating class of California, Texas and New York State,' she says. The problem is, she adds, that there's a belief in America that there is a way to make everything better, that everything can be fixed. 'And this has taken a destructive turn when applied to overweight people. Instead of working on making overweight people healthy and happy, society has decided that thinness is better, and out of that comes discrimination and prejudice and no celebration of human diversity. All efforts to lose weight involve some amount of self-hatred,' she continues. 'I would rather shed the self-hatred and not the weight. I have never dreamed of being in a thin body, but I have always dreamed of being treated with the same respect as my thin friends, and receiving the same opportunities,' she says. 'I just wish people would give up the false hope of being thin for the real hope of self-esteem.'

CHAPTER FIVE

IN SEARCH OF THE
MAGIC BULLET

'The likelihood that there will be a single magic bullet that's
going to be applicable to the treatment of the majority of
individuals with obesity is very, very unlikely.'

Doctor Rudy Leibel, Columbia University, New York

If dieting and keeping the pounds from piling back on requires such
hard work and commitment, it isn't hard to understand why
promises of a 'quick fix' can be very tempting. Whether it's a new
pill, a lotion you simply smooth on your skin, or a passive
body wrap, new products and treatments spring up regularly, are
widely advertised, and seduce us with promises of weight loss for
minimum effort.

Pills and Potions

One of the most high profile of these products to be launched recently is Fat Magnets, small capsules filled with matter extracted
from crushed lobster shells, produced by UK-based company
Swisshealth. John Langford, a manager with the company, explains
how they work. 'Fat Magnets is a chitosan-based product. Chitosan
is a naturally occurring shellfish fibre, which has the ability to
attract itself to fat.' It's a chemical reaction, he says. 'Fat is positively charged and chitosan is negatively charged,' and the chitosan
attracts fat like iron filings to a magnet, hence the product name.
'You take Fat Magnets just before you're going to eat your fattiest

meal of the day. They attract themselves to the fat molecules in the food before your digestive system gets it and stores it in places you don't want it to be stored,' he explains. This fat then passes away through normal bowel movements. 'You can in fact calculate the amount of fat that is removed by taking a stool and measuring the results.' Langford says this procedure has taken place during clinical trials. 'We invest heavily in research.' Fat Magnets, he claims, are currently the most successful aid to weight loss available.

Langford is quick to stress, however, that Fat Magnets are not a miracle pill. 'You don't just take these and eat as much as you like and not get fat. That is not what we profess to offer. People also need a diet, they need a lifestyle and they need a fitness programme. We give them every help we can.' Indeed, each tub of Fat Magnets comes with a sheet that gives diet and exercise advice. 'With Fat Magnets we have the ability to kick start people onto a programme. It's not a panacea to be a pig.'

When Fat Magnets first hit the market in 1996, says Langford, the response was remarkable. 'Over a four-day period we received 145,000 calls monitored by BT.' It was the first chitosan-based pill on the market at the time and, 'obviously it created a massive interest level.' Coverage in the media was widespread, but not all positive. 'There was quite an upsurge of cynicism about this new product,' admits Langford. This cynicism came not only from journalists, but also the medical profession. 'The response from doctors has been guarded. We've had one or two doctors be very, very critical of what we're doing.' Langford puts this down to annoyance at Fat Magnets stepping into their domain. 'I think they see themselves as the only source of a cure. They say that these naturally occurring substances, chitosan, Fat Magnets, are just another fad.'

Someone who agrees wholeheartedly with this view is John Garrow, Emeritus Professor of Nutrition at London's St Bartholomew's Hospital. Garrow is also Editor of the *European Journal of Clinical Nutrition* and Chairman of independent 'watchdog' organisation HealthWatch, through which he has conducted tests on chitosan-based slimming pills. 'They are not an effective weight loss remedy,' he states. 'The advertisements lead you to believe that if you take these capsules, which normally contain about 250 milligrams of chitosan each, before meals, they will bind with somewhere between 12 and 20 times their own weight in fat,' Garrow explains. As a result of this, the claim goes, you are unable to digest the fat, and so it passes out the other end. This suggests, Garrow adds, that you can therefore eat all the lovely fatty foods you want and still lose weight. 'This is not true.'

During the HealthWatch tests, Garrow measured the fat content of the stools of someone who had taken chitosan-based pills and compared it to someone who had not. 'In a normal person on a normal diet, the total amount of fat not absorbed, and therefore excreted in the stools, is about five grams a day.' So if someone was taking, for example, 3g. of chitosan a day, 1g. each at breakfast, lunch and dinner, and if each gram of chitosan bound to 12g. of fat as claimed, the tests should have detected an extra 36g. of fat in the stools of the person taking the pills. 'That is a huge amount,' says Garrow, 'and it would be terribly easy to detect. We found that there was no measurable change. That doesn't mean that there was no change,' he admits. 'There may have been an extra gram, because of course if you add any form of fibre to the diet, you get a slight increase in fat excretion, and chitosan comes under the heading of fibre. But then, you would do as well just eating wholemeal bread.'

Garrow points out that, this evidence aside, on theoretical grounds he would not expect such products to work. There are lots of instances in food preparation where it's convenient to have something that binds to fat; fat and flour, for example, need to bind together to make a cake. Garrow explains that chitosan will also bind with fat if the two are put together in a mixing bowl. However, he says, 'the human digestive system has always been very good at separating fats from other materials in food; that's what the digestive enzymes are there for. It is absurd to suppose that the feeble binding that occurs between chitosan and fat would actually defeat the human digestive system. It doesn't.'

Garrow isn't surprised, however, that these type of products – and there are several different brands of chitosan-based pills available – attract huge interest. People with weight problems can be vulnerable. 'There are an enormous number of wildly implausible claims made, and you think, "Surely no one is going to fall for that". But they do, and there are people who are making a lot of money out of totally useless weight loss remedies,' Garrow states. He points out that the only way to reduce the amount of body fat you have is to use up more energy than you take in, either by eating less or doing more exercise; and these conventional methods, while effective, are tedious. 'As a physician who's spent a lot of time trying to help severely obese patients, you realize that they can get pretty desperate. If someone has been ploughing away and has lost a stone or two, then suddenly they see this is all quite unnecessary, all they have to do is take some amazing pill, you can't blame them for thinking, "Let's give it a try",' he says. 'So they send off their money and get back a product which is totally useless.'

'We've never actually made a claim that [Fat Magnets] is 100 per cent successful for 100 per cent of the people, 100 per cent of the time,' says John Langford. He admits that some people have misunderstood how Fat Magnets are supposed to work, and used them as an excuse to overeat. 'If there's a misunderstanding and we have some responsibility for that, then I would immediately own up to that,' he says. 'We tell people how our products work, we're very open about who we are and what our products are made of. We're quite proud of what we do in the sense that we market a safe product and help people with a problem.' And, at the end of the day, 'If any client is not happy, of course we'll give them their money back.'

Garrow says that Langford's 'no guarantees' response is very wise. 'I'm glad he doesn't make guarantees. I just wish he'd make it more clear in his advertisements that he doesn't make guarantees, because the impression I have got from the them is that if you buy the stuff you can assume that you're one of the people for whom it will work,' he says. He adds that advertisements like this are often cleverly crafted and worded, and 'convey an impression which is untrue, without actually being untrue.' For example, companies may use before and after pictures depicting dramatic weight loss. These convey a certain impression and cause people to buy the product.

'When they get the product they open it up and in with the tub of pills will be something you unroll which is carefully worded, saying for example that this is terribly good in association with a calorie-controlled diet. So, for legal purposes obviously, statements are put into literature which you only see after you've parted with your money.' The company can then produce this in court, and claim that, if you look at the small print you'll see you need to diet as well. 'But that's not why people bought the product,' says Garrow. They thought they were getting a miracle pill. Garrow explains that these companies also use the 'money back guarantee' as insurance should they need to defend themselves. 'The point is that people who buy these products, and then find they are useless, are often so ashamed of themselves for having been conned that I presume they don't bother to claim their money back.'

Garrow explains that companies can get away with this sort of advertising because legislation is very poor. 'There are very strong laws for licensed prescription medicine. If you want to put a prescription medicine on the market you have to get a product license, and you've got to convince the Medicines Control Agency that what you're selling is pure, safe and effective.' Chitosan-based slimming pills, however, come under the umbrella of food or nutritional supplements or cosmetic aids, and different laws apply. 'You no more have to have a license than you do to sell cornflakes or scrambled eggs,' Garrow says. 'All that is necessary is for the manufacturer or advertiser to put out something that isn't actually poisonous, and they can more or less make any claim they like.'

However, if Trading Standards believes a company has made a false claim, they can bring a prosecution under the Trade Descriptions Act. Unlike prescription medicines, where the manufacturer has to prove their product works before they are able to sell it, the burden of proving a chitosan-based product, for example, does not work is on Trading Standards. And this is a lengthy process. 'The business of bringing these prosecutions is a tedious one,' says Garrow. Bringing a case might take nine months or a year. 'And by that time, the company involved might simply say, "Oh, terribly sorry, my goodness we made a mistake, we'll stop advertising this instant Your Honour". And the next week they'll start advertising the same material again but under a different name.'

Garrow points out that there are many other ineffective products and treatments on the market that tempt people as easy solutions. Creams that are rubbed into cellulite, ultrasound treatments and body wraps that claim to remove fat, for example, all do not work, he says. 'If any of these things worked it would be very important. Trials which showed they worked would be reported in all the scientific literature. They are not. If they really worked people like myself who have treated overweight patients on the NHS would use these techniques, but we don't.' Garrow also points out that theoretically, what these products claim to do is simply not possible.

'Fat is a material which sits in fat cells in a layer under the skin; it is not soluble in water. If by rubbing, or pummelling or ultra-sounding you managed to break it up and get it to go away, the only place it could go to would be into the bloodstream, and that would be very bad news.' He explains that droplets of fat in the bloodstream can occur when someone breaks a bone and as a result little bits of fatty marrow are released. 'This condition is called fat embolism. These little globules of fat move around in the blood until they come to a blood vessel that is too small for them to get through, and they block it up, causing damage. So,' he says, 'it's good news that these treatments don't work.' They are perfectly safe because, fortunately, they don't do what they claim.

Garrow explains that body wrap treatments which claim to reduce fat are also a con. 'If you get a bandage and wrap it quite tightly around a thigh, leave it there for a bit then take it off, the thigh will have got smaller. That is of course because the water has been squeezed out, and so you can alter the shape of a body part temporarily, but in 20 minutes or so it will be back to where it was before,' he says. 'None of these treatments affect the total amount of fat, which is the main problem.'

A *Health Which?* report released in February 1998 looked at 10 popular cellulite products and asked two leading dermatologists to comment on sales advice and product packaging claims. The report concluded that, "Expensive creams, lotions and oils bought in the hope of reducing the appearance of cellulite seem to be a waste of time and money". The independent research revealed that consumers could be taken in by misleading advice and a range of unsubstantiated, unrealistic or impossible claims. For example, many manufacturers claim that their products contain ingredients that will help shift fat, but *Health Which?* experts, and Professor Garrow, agree that there is no known substance which is proven to remove fat simply by being applied to the skin. In addition, none of the user trials which manufacturers offered as evidence of claims met *Health Which?* experts' standards for proving the products' effectiveness.

Garrow is angered by the presence of these treatments and their false promises. Overweight people can be very, very vulnerable, he says. He believes that one of the important reasons why obesity is such a serious public health problem in the United Kingdom and all over the world is that the conventional treatments available for it, 'are submerged in this great smokescreen of ridiculous magic cures. I mean, I don't much mind people making money dishonestly, but I do mind them reducing the ability of obese people to help themselves.'

Dr Susan Jebb of the Medical Research Council's Dunn Clinical Nutrition Centre agrees. 'Overweight people have often tried many times to lose weight, and very often, in the long run, have put it back on again and so feel they have failed.' And because they may not get the help and support they need from the established medical profession, she says, they can instead turn to alternative therapies. 'I'm extremely concerned because many of these are not proven to be effective for weight loss. Although as health professionals we tend to look at many of them and say, "Oh well, they're harmless", like a cream you rub in or a bath you sit in, in fact I'm not sure they are harmless. Anything that raises people's expectations but then lets them down actually perpetuates another cycle of failure. And I think that sets up a very pessimistic view for the future.'

Professor Philip James of the Rowett Research Institute feels society is to blame. 'There is an enormous amount of abuse going on in terms of the freedom in society to indulge in quackery, and the extraordinary claims that are made about weight loss.' The problem, he believes, is that the medical profession has not yet recognised that they have to take the problems of weight gain and obesity seriously. 'Until we get to a consensus amongst the medical establishment, we're not going to change government and cultural perceptions so that we get to the point where people won't be allowed to make outrageous claims, because they are misleading claims. There's not a piece of evidence that these sort of things help, and we are going to have to move towards a process that validates and regulates and analyses these claims, because they do an enormous amount of harm.'

Dr Catherine Steiner Adaire adds, 'There's a lot of misinformation about what health is, and there's a lot of preying on very vulnerable people by the weight loss industry,' she says, 'through the marketing of certain foods as being healthier than others, through miracle cure diets and miracle cure medicines. It's a huge problem, and the irony is that people are getting increasingly unhealthy, not more healthy.'

The Pharmaceutical War

At the moment, the fact remains that losing weight, for most of us, is hard work. Personal accounts of the struggle reveal that deprivation, hunger and misery are often never far out of the equation. A huge array of dietary products compete for the public's attention, assuring us that here, at last, is something that really works. Yet so many people are locked into the nightmare of yo-yo dieting. If only there was a simple, pain free solution. If only scientists would hurry up and produce a pill that would quickly and safely melt away excess body fat, getting rid of the need to slog away at diets and exercise programmes forever. The fact is, however, the pharmaceutical industry has so far only come up with drugs that work in a limited way, and often with dangerous side-effects.

According to the Obesity Research Information Centre (ORIC), the ideal anti-obesity drug would decrease appetite and increase energy expenditure, have no serious adverse effects and remain effective at producing medically useful weight loss throughout the time the medication was taken. This ideal, it points out, may be impossible to achieve. But that doesn't stop companies from trying. Most major pharmaceutical companies invest millions of pounds in the research and development of anti-obesity pills. The race to find the 'magic bullet' is well and truly under way. But is it really gaining any ground?

The use of drugs to aid slimming can be traced back to the 19th century, when a substance called ephedrine was extracted from a Chinese plant called *ephedra sinica* and consumed in tea as a stimulant. Using ephedrine and substances like it, scientists then developed amphetamines, a form of speed, which has an appetite-suppressant effect and were widely hailed in the 1960s as being the easy way to lose weight – until, that is, the side-effects became apparent. While amphetamines diminish feelings of hunger, they also stimulate the central nervous system, causing, among other things, increased blood pressure, heart palpitations, blurred vision, anxiety and insomnia. In addition, they can be addictive; because amphetamines produce a euphoric feeling, many became psychologically as well as physically addicted to them, and suffering terrible withdrawal symptoms, including black depression. Not only that, coming off these drugs caused increased appetite, and most people quickly gained back all the weight they had lost. Yet at the height of their popularity in the 1960s hundreds of thousands of people in Britain and the US were prescribed these pills; finally, by the mid-1960s, British doctors decided the problems associated with them were too great and voluntarily banned them.

Someone who knows well the effects of amphetamine-based pills is Professor Julia Polak, a senior pathologist at Hammersmith's Royal Postgraduate Medical School in London. In 1973 she took a three-month course of fenfluramine, an amphetamine-like appetite suppressant. The reason she took the pills, she says, is simple. 'Vanity. I wanted to look good in a bikini again after having a baby.' Actually, she says, she only had 1 or 2lb. to lose, and a little tummy bulge. But she took the pills and lost the weight, and had no idea of the consequences until 23 years later. 'I started to get very breathless,' she says. 'I thought it might have been asthma.' But in fact doctors diagnosed pulmonary hypertension and a failing heart. Three years ago Polak was given an emergency heart-lung transplant and two years to live. 'I believe I was born with a genetic predisposition for pulmonary hypertension,' she says, but thinks that taking fenfluramine contributed to the development of her life-threatening condition. 'Of course it is difficult to prove this now,' she says.

'The Royal College of Physicians sets down very clear guidelines for GPs in this country about prescribing slimming pills,' she adds. 'They should only be used in cases of extreme obesity and when all other treatments fail.' Polak believes that there is no way that taking fenfluramine for up to three months is safe. 'But individuals are affected differently, and of course not everybody who takes diet pills will develop pulmonary hypertension. There are genetics involved,' she says. 'Some people say that obesity is a major killer and it doesn't matter if a very small percentage of women die of pulmonary hypertension. Well for me, that percentage is 100 per cent.' Polak now lectures using specimens taken from her former heart and lungs, explaining the potential dangers of diet pills.

Since the 1960s, pharmaceutical companies have been churning out new pill after new pill, each being hailed as safer and more effective than the last. There are now many different types of pills being developed. In 1996, *Scientific American*, one of the world's leading science journals, published a study of 12 different slimming drugs in development, which fall into three main categories. First, drugs that act on the brain and reduce the signals we interpret as pangs of hunger (known as appetite suppressants); secondly, drugs that act on the digestive tract to either block fat from being absorbed or slow down the emptying of the stomach so that people feel full long; and thirdly, drugs that act on fat itself, to speed up fat burning.

In the United States many thousands of people were until recently prescribed a combination of two appetite-suppressant diet pills, known snappily as fen-phen: fenfluramine, which Professor Polak took, combined with phentermine. Although these drugs are chemically related to amphetamines, they work by increasing the amount of available serotonin, which regulates feelings of fullness. 1992 studies showed that if the drugs were taken together they would help dieters lose weight faster, and the combination rapidly became a hit. In 1996 alone 18 million prescriptions for fen-phen were written in the US, and many patients reported dramatic weight loss; the drug combination was not used in the UK. Sales hit hundred of millions of dollars and diet pill clinics sprang up all over the United States to capitalise on the euphoria. However, it wasn't to last.

In 1997, approximately four years after the combination first gained popularity, reports of serious side-effects hit the headlines. In July 1997 doctors at the Mayo Clinic in Rochester, Minnesota reported 24 cases of patients with heart valve damage which could be linked with fen-phen. The following month, the US Food and Drug Administration (FDA) reported 58 more cases of heart damage in users of the combination. Other fen-phen side-effects were reported to included pulmonary hypertension, brain damage and depression. In one widely reported case, a 29-year-old American woman developed pulmonary hypertension just 23 days after starting a course of fen-phen. Eight months later she was dead.

By September 1997 the makers of fenfluramine, Servier Laboratories, voluntarily withdrew the drug, one half of the combination, from sale. Although the FDA had approved the use of both fenfluramine and phentermine, the combination was never approved; this did not stop it being widely prescribed and easily available. When fenfluramine gained FDA approval in 1973, short-term use only was recommended, and it was meant only for severely obese patients who had tried other methods of treatment and failed, as Professor Polak points out. Phentermine is reported to be one of the most carefully tested diet pills on the market, and is still available in the US. However, although it is not addictive and has only mild side-effects, such as restlessness and constipation, it is reported to have only a moderate success rate.

Another popular appetite suppressant, dexfenfluramine, marketed as Redux in the US and Adifax in the UK, was withdrawn in the States at the same time as fen-phen, and subsequently taken off the market in the UK; currently, there are no pharmaceutical drugs in the UK specifically for the treatment of obesity. Dexfenfluramine works in the same way as fenfluramine, and was found to have similar side-effects. In fact, the FDA was said to have received unconfirmed reports of about 1,000 adverse reactions to Redux in the first two million prescriptions; these reactions included 18 deaths and 26 'serious psychiatric events'. It was the only anti-obesity drug licensed in the UK for use for more than 12 weeks, but not more than one year; when it got FDA approval in the US it passed with no restrictions on the period of use. Now it has been deemed too dangerous for use at all. America is renowned for its lawsuit mentality, and already there has been a rash of damages cases across the country following the withdrawal of both drugs. Some experts are predicting the Redux/fenfluramine recall could turn into one of the biggest medical liability cases ever.

Yet another new drug development is known as orlistat, marketed as Xenical, which works to block the absorption of fat rather than suppress the appetite. A one-year trial on 4,000 patients showed that it can cut out about 600 calories a day, with an average annual weight loss of 1st. 7lb. The bad news is that the undigested fat must be excreted, and reported side-effects include diarrhoea and 'anal leakage', which gets worse as more fat is eaten. Xenical is still waiting for FDA approval in the US, and experts believe it could shortly be available both in the US and Europe.

The newest development of all is a drug called sibutramine, which is sold in the US as Meridia; it increases the feeling of fullness, and studies on animals show it may also enhance metabolic rate, speeding up the burning of fat. Trials have shown that it seems to work mainly in the brain. It got FDA approval in early 1998, and was only recently launched in the US. It is not yet available in the UK, and only time will tell how safe it really is.

Dr Rudy Leibel, Professor of Medicine & Paediatrics at New York's Columbia University, says the diet pills currently used are a long way off being the magic bullet so many people hope for. 'They are cannon balls, shot at people's heads,' he says. 'They use a sledgehammer approach to the problem of obesity.' He likens taking these pills to shooting yourself in the head in an effort to get rid of a headache. 'That will relieve the headache in the sense that I won't be feeling anything any more, but it's a very drastic form of treatment if you consider that what you're really aiming for is a very specific pharmacologic effect.' In other words, while many of the diet drugs available are to help people lose weight, that isn't all they do; they are not that targeted. They reduce weight, but at the risk of enormous damage elsewhere in the body, as these recent cases have graphically illustrated. Leibel believes that pharmaceutical companies are acting in the best faith when they release these drugs. 'The pharmaceutical companies, the scientists, are trying to design drugs that are effective at producing weight reduction. It turns out, very unfortunately, that these have had very severe side-effects which weren't immediately appreciated when the drugs were developed.'

And despite the myriad of different pills available and those in development, and the huge amount of money drugs companies sink into research, Leibel believes the 'magic bullet' is still a long way off. 'Sibutramine is a next-generation drug in the sense that the side-effects are likely to be less severe, or somewhat muted, but nonetheless, there are going to be side-effects. Hopefully these are not going to be of the severity we've seen in the fen-phen case,' he continues, 'and we have no reason to expect that at this time, but sibutramine does not represent a sea change or a quantum leap in terms of sophisticated pharmacology with regard to the treatment of obesity.' Leibel says it's simply an evolutionary step, not a revolutionary one.

'Sibutramine will definitely cause changes in blood pressure in some patients; this is already a known side-effect of that drug, and I'm sure the drug will also be monitored for some of the side-effects that have now been appreciated with regard to fenfluramine. However,' Leibel adds, 'that doesn't mean there won't be new side-effects as well, side effects that haven't been detected before.' Although he says sibutramine may well assist in the treatment of obesity in some people, what is really needed is for scientists to keep trying to understand the physiology of weight reduction and how the body regulates, or fails to regulate, its weight. Only then, ultimately, can very targeted drugs that address very specific aspects of metabolism or food intake without affecting other parts of the body, be developed. 'However, the likelihood that there will be a single magic bullet that's going to be applicable to the treatment of the majority of individuals with obesity is very, very unlikely,' he concludes.

Yale University's Professor Kelly Brownell agrees. 'We need safe and effective medications to help overweight people, but I don't think any medication will ever come along that will wipe out the obesity problem,' he says. 'The medications that we have at our disposal now produce modest weight losses, and people tend to maintain the weight loss as long as they're on the medication.' So they become part of the answer to the problem, but only part. 'They are something that physicians can offer to the overweight person but they are not a solution to the obesity problem,' he explains. 'Scientific studies show that people who go off these weight loss medications tend to regain their weight. And we, the public and the field, have viewed that as a sign that the medication is a failure,' he says. However, Brownell believes obesity should be viewed as a chronic, or long-term, condition which requires long-term treatment. 'Then the fact that people regain weight when the medicine is discontinued is evidence that it's working. It just argues for keeping people on medication for a long time, as would be the case if somebody had diabetes or hypertension or chronic heart disease.'

Brownell says only time will tell whether new medications like sibutramine have been tested for long enough before coming on the market. 'It's possible that some health consequences will be apparent but only after a longer period of time than they have been tested for.'

He points out that the FDA in the United States and regulatory agencies in other countries have to decide a point at which they feel new medications are safe enough, given their benefits, to release onto the market. 'My fervent hope is that more and more medications will come on the market, that they will become safer as time goes on, with fewer side-effects and have greater weight losses, because people desperately need something to help them.'

CHAPTER SIX

FIT & FAT

'We simply do not need to obsess about our weight. Human beings, after all, come in various sizes and shapes, and some of us are always going to be short and stocky and others tall and skinny. What we need to do is accept what we are and focus on what we can do to be healthy.'

Dr Steven Blair,
Cooper Institute for Aerobics Research, Dallas

Fifty-three-year-old Dave Alexander is 5ft. 8in. tall, weighs 250lb. and is classified as morbidly obese; he is more than 7st. over the weight range recommended in the medical charts for a man of his height. Many people in the medical profession would consider him to be in the danger zone, and at high risk of developing conditions like diabetes, hypertension and heart disease. But Dave isn't worried. In fact, he considers himself to be superbly healthy. 'In an average week I swim five miles, run 30 miles and do about 200 miles of cycling,' he says. Since 1983 he has completed 265 triathlons in places as far afield as China, Germany, Malaysia, Turkey and the United States. He is, he says, a fit, active, healthy man who also happens to be fat. 'I'm healthy, I feel good, and I could get up and run a marathon right now.'

According to the charts, Dave has always been overweight. 'I weighed 214 pounds and was 5 feet 8 inches when I was 12 years old. I've been heavy my whole life. I also have a very large bone structure. One doctor said that my hips would fit on a 7-foot man.' However, although his health and fitness improved greatly when he began exercising, Dave's weight and shape has hardly changed. 'It doesn't seem to matter how much I eat or how much I exercise; my weight stays fairly constant. It'll go up and down a little bit, but not very much.' So why, when he does more hard aerobic exercise than most people, does he find it so difficult to lose weight? The problem, Dave believes, revolves around his metabolism.

'My metabolism is unusual,' he explains. 'It is normal, like most people's, when I'm up and moving around, but when I'm sedentary it drops very quickly.' Dave points to the fact that as soon as he stops moving, he gets very cold. 'It's very warm here in Phoenix, but even in the summer time I have to sleep with blankets over me. It's because my metabolic rate drops so much when I'm resting.' Normally, he says, a person's metabolic rate drops very slowly after exercise. 'If they could raise my resting metabolic rate, I would lose a lot of weight very fast.'

Dave admits that he would indeed like to be able to lose some weight, but says he would never be able to weigh within the range recommended by the charts; that is, between 130 and 165 pounds, between 9 and a half and 11 and a half stone. 'That would be impossible for my body type. My total lean body mass weighs more than that,' Dave says. In other words, tests have shown that his muscle and bones alone weigh more than his recommended weight. So the doctors have, Dave believes, got it wrong. 'Everyone's different and I think the range for what is healthy is much broader than they will admit.' People, he says, are simply built differently. 'I don't think it's possible to have one chart that fits everybody on the entire planet.'

Dave Alexander's doctor, Craig Phelps, agrees. 'There are some people who defy the normal descriptions of fitness and what's healthy,' he says; people like Dave, who don't conform to the recommendations in height/weight tables. 'And these are people who shouldn't be made to feel bad because they are overweight. We need to acknowledge their fitness and health levels and use them as a model and a positive influence for other people.' Dr Phelps has put Dave though rigorous tests and found, initially to his surprise, that the 250-pound man is terribly healthy. 'His resting pulse is in the 60s, like a trained athlete; his blood pressure is usually in the 120s over 80s, which again for most people is a very normal blood pressure. We've exercised him to the point of exhaustion on the treadmill many times, checking for any cardiac abnormalities, and everything we've detected to date shows that he is fit, except for his weight.'

A Broader View

What this tells us, Phelps says, is that there are some people out there who defy the normal description of fitness and what's healthy. 'This is telling us is that we have to step back and look at people individually. Dave is certainly a perfect example of this. He's overweight, but he's fit. He is one of those unique individuals who is off the charts.' In the past, he says, we've tried to get overweight people to conform to a weight level that the medical profession considers healthy, or to a weight that looks 'right'. The problem is, however, that many people were simply not designed to get to those weight levels. 'If Dave got down to between 130 and 165 pounds he'd really be starving himself to death. He certainly wouldn't be fit or able to perform at the level he does now,' Phelps says.

However, he also points out that people like Dave are not that common. 'The population of Phoenix for instance is about two million people, and Dave is probably one in two million who can do what he does, yet look like he does. His body is very big, very strong, but he has some endurance capabilities that most people don't have. There are probably seven Daves in Los Angeles and seven Daves in London, and these people could no more get down to the ideal weight than most 'normal' weight people could walk around at 600 or 700 pounds and survive.' But people like this, he says, should help us realise there is a wide variation in what is healthy. 'When we run across these people on rare occasions, they serve as models for the rest of us.'

Phelps believes there are two main reasons that Dave finds it so hard to lose weight, despite the amount of exercise he does. 'Number one, he has a unique metabolism. There's no doubt about this. He can go out and expend a tremendous amount of effort in a race, but drop very few pounds. Someone else participating in these activities might lose 5, 10, 15 pounds. Dave doesn't. So I think there's an inborn metabolism switch which he has, and the majority of us don't have.' The second reason for Dave's weight, though, according to Phelps, is his diet. 'I think Dave still, on occasion, tends to eat more than he should, and that's part of his personality. He goes after everything with gusto and although he tries to control his diet, I think he can improve on that.' If he was a little more vigilant with his diet, Phelps says, he would drop some weight. 'I think there's room for Dave to come down on his overall body fat, but certainly not to the extreme weight recommended in the charts.'

The Dangerous Ideal

Dr Phelps, who as well as running his own practice, is also team doctor for the Arizona Ballet, believes that people have an image of the perfect body weight for them based on what society decides is the ideal. 'Looking at weight in a cosmetic sense is extremely dangerous.' Instead, he says, if people focused more on health and fitness rather than the cosmetic, weight would probably take care of itself. 'Then there's less tendency for weight to yo-yo and fluctuate, and people begin to focus more on the positive aspects.' He admits, though, that this is hard to do in a society which rates body image as a very important part of overall identity.

'Throughout the world, but especially in the developed countries, society is very visually oriented,' says Phelps. We constantly see images of the 'ideal', which are considered healthy and beautiful, on television, in magazines, and in the performing arts. 'But take someone like a ballet dancer or a star basketball or soccer player. These people have spent hours a day, years of their lives perfecting what they do and as a result they've developed a body or a physique that is fairly unattainable for the average person,' he points out. 'Ballet dancers, for example, are often in class six hours a day, sometimes even longer, and they're burning a tremendous number of calories.'

Sometimes, he says, the pressure they are under can actually cause ballet dancers to overdo it in pursuit of physical perfection. 'Not only do they have to exercise and perform many hours a day, they also have to look a certain way.' And that look is something which is, for the average person and the majority of the population, impossible to get to. 'So you have a ballet dancer who is not only working hard and prone to injury, but is also trying to maintain this almost mythological appearance, and these factors can sometimes lead to both mental and physical problems.' Not only can dancers develop injuries resulting from over-exercising, but eating disorders such as anorexia and bulimia can occur.

Moderation, stresses Phelps, is the key. 'The more we deal with people, the more we know that if they maintain a moderate course they usually do pretty well.' A lot of people, he says, are worrying unnecessarily about their weight for cosmetic reasons, and really need to embrace the idea of being as fit and healthy as they can. 'When people do this, the emotional pressure is off and the weight tends to take care of itself.' But forget trying to look like the current ultra-slim ideal, he says. 'In fact, you can attain that look yet be very unfit and unhealthy.'

The Height/Weight Tables: Is There Really an Ideal?

The height/weight tables used by the medical profession today were actually developed by insurance companies back in the 1950s, as a way of categorizing people and assessing the risks of over-weight in relation to life insurance claims. Many experts today believe they are not only biased, but outmoded and too rigid. 'The ideal body weight tables have come from life insurance companies, pure and simple. They have not been intelligently put together by doctors,' says Dr Andrew Prentice of the Dunn Clinical Nutrition Centre. 'I think doctors do need to wise up to this, and to look at their patients in a much more holistic way.' Instead of simply making judgements based on a person's weight, doctors should, he says, consider each individual and their overall state of health. 'There is no doubt that the medical profession's use of height/weight guidelines as applicable to everyone has oversimplified things,' Prentice says.

Dr Rudy Leibel of New York's Columbia University agrees, and believes that everyone has their own, individual 'ideal' weight range. Studies, he says, have shown that there is a perfectly acceptable wide variation of weights for different people. 'And high levels of body fat are not necessarily associated with bad health, just as low levels of body fat are not necessarily associated with good health.' If a person is overweight but doesn't have any of the conditions that are often associated with obesity and overweight – high blood pressure, diabetes, degeneration of joints, for example – in other words is healthy, that is what matters. 'That's a pretty good piece of evidence that they are at their normal and acceptable degree of body fatness, and should probably be left alone,' he says.

Yale University's Professor Kelly Brownell feels that height/weight tables are really just another factor putting pressure on overweight people. 'The problem with the tables of ideal weight,' he says, 'is that they hold out a specific number as the perfect level to attain, and people feel they have to get to that level in order to have made progress.' Instead, he believes, people should be encouraged to attain a healthier weight, rather than an 'ideal' one. 'We're so caught up in this idea that overweight is the person's fault, that their body shape and weight are under personal control and that the only thing that lies between an individual and the perfect body is personal effort.'

Brownell feels that the ideal weight charts are as counter-productive to society as the beauty ideals that many people aspire to. 'It may be ideal from a health point of view to have a BMI of 24, but it's totally unrealistic for people living in the real world. I advocate very strongly getting rid of the beauty ideals, and I think getting rid of the health ideals would help too.' Just losing a small amount of weight is good, he says. 'Some impressive health benefits can come from relatively modest weight losses, such as five or 10 per cent of initial body weight. I try to convince people that even if they only lose a small amount of weight, which to them may seem cosmetically insignificant, it could have important health benefits. So it's not a question of attaining an ideal, it's a question of doing the best you can.'

Great Shape

'For years I was virtually the only large woman in sight at any gym or exercise class I attended,' says Kathryn Szrodecki, a YMCA-certified exercise instructor who runs fitness classes for large women. Through talking to big women, she discovered two main reasons many feel unable to exercise. 'Firstly, they often feel out of place and unwelcome in an exercise environment, and secondly, if they do make it into a gym or class, they are required to do exercises unsuitable for people their size,' Kathryn explains.

Larger women, she says, have often found themselves at high risk of injury in the average class; the larger body moves and responds differently to that of an average-sized person. 'And most instructors tell participants to go at their own pace, but the larger exerciser feels self-conscious enough being the only big woman in the room. She won't take the risk of standing out even more by doing less than the rest of the class.'

Tired of feeling like this herself, Kathryn decided to do something about it. She started a company called Alternative Size, and produced an exercise video, Great Shape, designed specifically for large women. 'I want to show that exercise is for everyone, irrespective of size.' She also runs weekly fitness classes in London and has a very enthusiastic following. 'But until fitness instructors are trained to cater for all body sizes within a gym or class, and to place less emphasis on an ideal body shape,' she says, 'it seems inevitable that most fitness environments will remain dangerous and unwelcoming places, and therefore 'off limits' to large women.'

The Fitness Factor

Like many others, Dr Steve Blair of the Cooper Institute for Aerobics Research in Dallas, Texas, believes we have created an environment in which it is virtually impossible for people who are genetically susceptible to obesity to avoid it. 'There are too many opportunities to be sedentary. We've engineered physical activity out of existence. On top of that you have immediate access to food, and it's cheap. For someone like me, it's virtually impossible to overcome the problem,' he says. As well as conducting research into the relationship between weight and health, Blair is a dedicated runner.

'I have run nearly every day for the last 30 years. I religiously do about 35 miles a week,' he says. 'I think I've probably run three times around the world.' He exercises, eats well, is fit and healthy, and he also happens to have a body mass index (BMI) of over 30; in other words he is obese and, according to conventional medicine, in the danger zone for illness and early death. 'But I consider myself fat and fit,' Blair says. 'I think I'm probably very well suited to life as a serf on the Russian steppes. I am strong, I can work hard, and in earlier times I would have been quite successful in surviving the famines that were inevitable. Now, there haven't been many famines in North Dallas in recent times, and even though I exercise regularly and try to eat a healthful diet, my energy expenditure level overall is still low by historical and evolutionary standards.' Quite simply, he says, 'I'm not well suited to being a scientist leading an essentially sedentary life, onto which I graft this artificial dose of exercise every day.'

But while obesity or overweight may be hard for many to avoid, there is some good news. Blair has conducted an eight-year study, involving 25,000 men, which examined the relationship between weight and health. 'We measured the cardio-respiratory fitness and calculated the body mass index of these men, then followed them for eight years,' he explains. 'Surprisingly, we found that the men who were fat but also fit actually had no increased mortality rate. In fact, the fat and fit men had far lower death rates than the 'normal' rate men who were unfit. So the bottom line in this research is that lack of fitness seems to be much more important than fatness as a predictor of which men were going to die during the eight-year follow up.'

Blair adds, however, that it would be wrong to dismiss totally the idea that excessive body fat is a health hazard. People who are very obese and very sedentary are in a dangerous position. 'It's very difficult to draw a precise line and say, "If you're on this side you are so obese that it's a medical emergency",' he says. 'But I think that when people get to a BMI above 35 or 40, it does become a serious medical condition.' However, he points out, 'We have tens of millions of people who are only moderately overweight, say by 20, 30, even 50 pounds, and that's a different matter.' It deserves attention, he says, but is something that eating healthily and exercising can help enormously.

While some may view the notion that it's possible to be fit and fat as quite revolutionary, Blair sees it simply as a positive message. 'I think it's actually a good news public health message, because we have a lot of people who are overweight by the conventional criteria, and many of them are unsuccessful in losing weight and keeping it off. So, I'm trying to give the positive message that there's something you can do. You can exercise regularly, you can improve your physical fitness and greatly improve your health status, and in doing so lower your risk of premature mortality.'

A Healthy Balance

Blair also agrees that standardizing weight too rigidly is a problem. 'I think we all have a weight range at which we can be healthy and functional and happy in life, and this,' Blair believes, 'is determined largely by our inheritance. We shouldn't focus too much on a single number and we certainly should not assume that it's the same number for different individuals.' The claim that some formula can produce a so-called 'ideal' weight that can then be applied to an individual, is, he says, faulty logic.

In addition, Blair feels the medical profession has focused too much attention on obesity and overweight, and not enough on the effects of low levels of exercise and fitness. 'I think we need to address the balance a little more and we need to encourage activity more.' Indeed, he says, many overweight or obese people are unhealthy mainly because they don't exercise. 'And I think lack of activity, low levels of energy expenditure, is the predominant cause of obesity in our society.'

However, Blair points out that while exercise doesn't affect weight very much in the short-term, lack of exercise can add up over time. 'I think it can have a tremendous effect on weight over the long-term, over the years and decades.' He points out that even a small excess of calories a day builds up over time. 'But it's very hard to take off very many pounds by exercise. The general rule of thumb is that 35 miles of walking take off one pound of fat. On the other hand, if I weren't doing my 35 miles of running a week, I would be gaining a pound a week, and that's about 50 pounds a year.' So, he says, the accumulation of exercise can be incredibly important in maintaining or preserving body weight, or slowing the rate of weight gain over time. 'Or even gradually losing weight. It just doesn't happen quickly.'

Like others, Blair too is frustrated by the presence of extreme beauty ideals. 'Just disabuse yourself of this notion of the ideal stick-thin model,' he says. 'We have these impossible ideals that people aspire to, whether it's models or movie stars or, God forbid, Barbie. I mean, there's probably not one woman in 10 million who can have Barbie's proportions, even if they use cosmetic surgery and starve themselves and exercise regularly. I mean, it's an impossibility.' We simply do not need to obsess about our weight, he says. 'Human beings, after all, do come in various sizes and shapes, and some of us are always going to be short and stocky and others tall and skinny.' What we need to do is accept what we are and focus on what we can do to be healthy, he says.

Banish the Scales

'Eat a healthful diet, exercise regularly, enjoy the things that life has to offer, and don't obsess so much about the number on the scales.' This, Blair stresses, is crucial. 'There are millions of people who every day get up and step on the scales, and they let the scales tell them whether it's going to be a good day or a bad day. If they're up a pound they say, "Oh, isn't this terrible, I don't know what I've done wrong", but if they're a pound down they say, "I must be doing something right". That's silly,' he states. 'It's an unpleasant way to live if you're constantly fretting about every single ounce. As enthusiastic as I am about exercise, frankly I get a little bored with people who want to talk about nothing but their exercise programme and the time of their last 10 kilometre run.' After all, he says, there's so much more to enjoy in life.

'In America we spend tens of billions of dollars a year in the pursuit of thinness, and yet we're progressively getting fatter,' states Blair. It is clear, therefore, that haranguing people into losing weight isn't working. Like many others, he suggests changing the environment so that greater activity and less consumption of junk food are encouraged. 'We need new strategies, like making our cities more liveable,' he says. 'For example, by banning automobile traffic in certain parts of the city so you have to walk, and making it safe and pleasant to go outside and be physically active.' People should simply be encouraged to get out and move around. 'Cycle, skateboard, walk, jog, do whatever they like.' And hopefully without getting anxious and obsessive. 'I think we should be relaxed. I think we should strive for a healthful diet, but I don't think we should try to follow a bunch of rigid rules and obsess about everything we do. To me it's really very simple. A lot of fruit and vegetables, a lot of whole grains and not too much fat or alcohol.' And, of course, regular exercise. Blair suggests starting to walk even short distances, then accumulating to between 30-45 minutes a day. 'By doing these things, your weight will probably go down and be more where you would like it to be.'

Weight and Health

Studies worldwide have shown that some of the conditions linked to obesity include coronary heart disease, diabetes, and certain forms of cancer, all of which can lead to premature death. Infertility in women, osteoarthritis and joint problems, respiratory difficulties and depression have also been linked to overweight and obesity. The medical costs of obesity have been estimated to be between four to six per cent of the health costs of affluent countries. 'In the UK, with the health budget exceeding £40 billion, this would amount to between £1.6 and £2.4 billion pounds a year,' says Dr Andrew Prentice of the Dunn Clinical Nutrition Centre. Studies suggest that the more weight a person gains, and therefore the higher their BMI gets, the greater their chance of developing health problems.

Words of Caution

Although many experts agree it is possible for people to be both fat and fit, this is certainly not always the case. 'The evidence is quite strong that there are a few people, and I stress a few people, who in spite of being very, very overweight are very fit,' says Dr Andrew Prentice. But, he stresses, they are a rarity. 'I think it's rather dangerous to suggest it's okay to be fat, and really it's fitness that counts. We know this is not the case. There is no doubt that being overweight is a significant indicator of premature mortality.' This, he adds, has been proven in study after study. 'We know that obesity is more likely to cause someone to die young than if they're leaner. And we know many fat people suffer an enormous amount of misery because they're grossly debilitated from living a normal life.'

However, he says, it is very important to tease out those overweight or obese people who are at greatest risk. 'And not tell every fat person they're in danger of dying tomorrow, because that's not true.' Some patients, he says, will be very overweight and yet very, very healthy. 'And they are probably best left well alone. I think we have created an enormous amount of damage by castigating all fat people.'

Professor Kelly Brownell agrees that it is possible for people who are overweight by health standards to be fit, if they are doing a lot of physical activity. 'But the same could be said of smokers. You could find a smoker who doesn't seem to suffer any health consequences and lives to 102,' he says. 'Just because you have exceptions to the rule, doesn't change the rule that being overweight is unhealthy.'

Dr Susan Jebb, however, points out that there are people who, according to the tables, are overweight but not *over fat*. 'The classic example is athletes who are extremely muscular. They may be heavy but they are not fat, and clearly they do not have the same health risks as a person who is overweight and over fat,' she explains. However, she believes that physical activity and fitness can actually help to protect against some of the dangers of overweight. 'Whether it actually obliterates those dangers is very controversial,' she admits. But, she adds, physical activity certainly helps to reduce the health risks of obesity.

CHAPTER SEVEN
THE FAT PRACTICE

> 'I have a war on obesity because of the gross prejudice, because of the extreme unfairness in our society towards the obese. They're being treated as the modern equivalent of lepers, and I'm a leper doctor.'
>
> *Dr George Cowan, Obesity Surgeon,*
> *University of Tennessee, Memphis*

Twenty-four-year-old Christie Martin lives with her husband and five-year-old daughter Olivia in a small town in the American state of Arkansas. Christie is classified as morbidly obese; she weighs just over 500lb. and is, she says, slowly and painfully dying. Christie was heavy as a very young child and has suffered the physical, emotional and social consequences of being overweight all her life. 'I couldn't wait to start school,' she remembers. As a little girl she would often go to meet her older sister as she arrived home on the bus. 'I'd be grinning from ear to ear, jumping up and down and yelling, "Here comes the school bus!" So on my first day of school I remember finally stepping on that bus, grinning, with my new backpack on, and as soon as I got to the top step all the kids immediately called out, "We got us a butterball this year". That was my nickname from then on, and every morning they'd go, "Butterball, butterball".' She was just five years old.

When Christie got to school that first day, she met another little girl and thought she'd found her first friend. 'We just hit it off, but then all the other kids started whispering, and the next thing I knew, my new friend said, "I can't be your friend because you're fat".' Within her first two hours of school, Christie says, her joy was shattered. 'All my anticipation and expectations were shot. I went out to the playground and I was alone, and it hit me then that there was something wrong with me. I'd never imagined before that there was anything wrong with me.'

And so began the struggle of a lifetime. Christie's parents, worried about her weight, started to restrict her food intake and encourage her to exercise, both of which, Christie believes, made the problem worse. 'Mum would only put a little bit of food on my plate, but everyone else could eat as much as they liked. Even at that young age they would say things like, "You're going to get as big as a house", and everyone watched every bite I put in my mouth.' While Christie's mum was in charge of her eating, her father looked after the exercise side. 'My dad would have me out in the evening running laps around our yard, and I did a hundred sit-ups every night. By the time I was nine or 10 years old I was enrolled in an adult aerobics class; I had to do aerobics every day after school, a child in with a bunch of adults.' All of this simply made Christie feel even more different from everyone else. 'We'd go to see the doctor about my weight, and that night for supper I'd have half a tuna salad sandwich on my plate, and everybody else had fried potatoes, fried chicken and gravy, a big, old southern meal. I would just choke that sandwich down. It really hurt me that I couldn't have what everyone else had.'

This, Christie believes, led her to develop an obsession with food. 'When it came time to clear the table, I'd be in the kitchen making sure no one was looking and I'd grab whatever was left over, because I was just really hungry. I don't know if it was because I was really, really hurt that I was being treated so harshly and food was made to be such an issue, or if it was a psychological problem I was having. But food became an issue 24 hours a day, and I felt like I had to sneak when I wanted something to eat.'

As time went on and Christie steadily got bigger, she tried almost everything to lose weight. 'I've been on different weight loss programmes. I've been bulimic, making myself sick every time I ate. I've tried crash dieting and counting fat grams and carbohydrate grams and starving myself. I've done it all. I've been on several different diet pills, and they would help me lose weight, but they would either elevate my blood pressure or I would have other side-effects, like mood swings and depression, and the doctor would pull me off them.' The awful thing, Christie says, is that the more she worried about her weight and food, the worse things got. 'The more I worried about how people were going to treat me, the more I stayed inside. Then you tend to eat more, you sit around, you worry, you feel sorry for yourself, you cry, you eat and it all makes it even worse. I'd think, "I shouldn't have eaten that", and then I'd get depressed and feel like a failure.' It is, she says, a vicious circle.

Christie was obese when she gave birth to her daughter Olivia five years ago, and she has never felt able to be the mother she wants to be. While she finds if difficult enough to cope with every-day life, it is her inability to give her daughter what she needs that really breaks Christie's heart. 'Everything I want to do I have to think about well ahead of time. I have to really limit the things Olivia can do, and that hurts me and it bothers her. Sometimes she'll make a comment like, "Well, I'll just get a new mummy", and she's joking with me, but it makes me wonder sometimes if that's maybe what she needs,' Christie says sadly. 'There is so much Olivia needs and wants, and the most I can give her is my love. I do things with her, but not what the other parents are doing with their children, and she'll say that to me. She's only five years old, but she knows there's a difference.'

Christie is terribly afraid that people will make judgements about Olivia because her mother is overweight. 'Olivia loves me very much, and I don't think she thinks about it, but I do. I think she's so special and beautiful and she's got so much personality, and I'm afraid that if people see that I'm her mum, they're going to pass judgement on her. I want people to see her for who she is and not to judge her because she's got a great big fat mamma. But people do.' Little children of Olivia's age already make comments at school, says Christie. 'So I don't go to her school any more. I just drive her there and drop her off. I did walk her in a few times, but she would tell me later what other children had said. She'd come home and say, "Mummy, are you fat?" or "So and so said you've got a really big belly, Mummy".' Christie began to feel so worried and ashamed that she now asks friends or her mother to accompany Olivia to school events. 'With other kids making comments like that to her, I guess I'm afraid that she's going to end up feeling the same way about me.'

This is just one of many issues Christie has to cope with as she goes about her life. Everyday activities that most of us take for granted can also be difficult obstacles for her. 'Regular household activities seem to take so much out of me. I've had people say, "Oh, that's because you're lazy", but I'll have 101 things planned to do, and once I start doing them I just run out of energy,' she explains. 'The biggest hang-up I have is just running small errands. This is not a physical thing, it's a mental thing,' she says quietly. 'I just don't want to go out of the house, because then I have to deal with the public. Some people are really great, but the majority just stare at me or are rude to me, or they just ignore me like I'm not even there.'

Experience has taught Christie that, for her, going out into the world can be dangerous. 'One Friday night Olivia and I went to a department store that's right next to the movie theatre in our town,' she explains. 'There was a group of teenagers standing in line to buy tickets, and when we walked past after shopping they saw me and cried out and got everybody's attention. There was this whole group of people there, and every step I took on the way to my car, I heard them going, "Boom-bubba, boom-bubba", the whole way to my car.' Christie tried to get into the car as quickly as possible, but already Olivia had started to ask what was going on. 'She said, "Mummy, why are they doing that? Why are they doing it?"' By this time, Christie was crying. 'Olivia asked why, and I just didn't want to tell her that they were making fun of me. I won't ever forget that.'

And that same night, as Christie and Olivia drove home, a car full of teenagers pulled up beside them and stayed with them all the way home. 'They were making slurs, making fun of me and saying, "You're too fat to drive". How could they do that in front of my kid? She means so much to me, and I just don't want her to be affected by me being this way.'

Incidents like this are common for Christie. She tells another agonizing story. 'I went to a grocery store one day to get a couple of things, and the lines were really backed up. Suddenly, this child said, "Look mummy, a great big fat person", and everybody just burst out laughing. I'm not exaggerating, just about everybody in those lines, even the check-out people, turned around to look at me. Olivia was waiting for me in the car, and the only thing I could think was, "I'm so glad Olivia did not hear this".' Christie is astounded by how ignorant and cruel people can be. 'If my child had said something like that, made a comment about someone, I would pull her aside and say, "God made people different. Just because someone's different, you don't tease them. You love them for who they are".'

A lifetime of feeling ostracised and alone has left Christie a broken and unhappy woman. 'I feel like I've just been a failure, that I haven't done things right. I can't have done things right because I look the way I do and I am the way I am. I just feel like I've been a failure at everything,' she says sadly. 'I'm afraid of the constant rejection in my life. I can't handle it any more. You know, I don't have one mirror in my house that shows more than my face, because I hate looking at myself. It's like I'm someone else trapped in this body. I'm suffocating in this body.' But Christie admits she makes things even harder for herself. 'I feel guilty all the time. If Olivia's having a bad day I feel guilty, I automatically feel it's my fault. And there's this little person in my head that says, "God you're so ugly, you're so fat, you're a failure, a slob, you're lazy". I am really hard on myself.'

The overriding feeling Christie gets from the outside world, however, is that she has let herself get this way because she simply doesn't care. 'I don't care enough, apparently, or I wouldn't have got to this point. But I do care, I care a great deal.' Society, she says, treats you like an outcast if you're overweight. 'People make you feel worse than you already do about yourself. It makes you start to live like a hermit, locked in a dark room. It hurts so bad to be socially unacceptable. All my life I've been treated like that and I've actually started to believe it. I am at the point in my life where I don't believe that anyone could possibly love me, and if they say they love me I don't trust them. Why would you love someone who looks like me?' she asks. The one place Christie knows she is loved, however, is her church. 'The people there do love me, and they have no hesitations about me. They accept me for exactly who I am, and that's really important to me.'

Despite this one place of acceptance, Christie has clearly reached a point where she feels defeated and frightened by her condition. 'I know it's not cancer, and I know it's not Alzheimer's or anything like that, but I'm slowly watching the weight take me over. Something I could do last week I might not be able to do this week or next week. It's like a gradual breakdown and I'm seeing it happen, and it scares me,' she admits. 'It's very depressing, and you need to have a positive attitude, but it's so hard to stay positive when everything hurts and everything's difficult, and you not only feel physical pain, but you feel emotional pain. You know, it's just very hard to deal with.'

After years of misery, years of trying but failing to lose weight, and years of being treated unsympathetically by doctors, Christie has decided to take drastic action. She is going to have obesity surgery. In fact, she believes this is her last chance. 'If I don't have this operation, I will definitely die. That's what's going to happen, according to the doctors I've seen.' There are days, she says, when she actually feels her life slipping away. 'I call them my bad days.

I've just got to the point where everything is hard. Sleeping, driving, walking, everything is difficult.' Christie knows that the operation itself involves risk. 'I'm afraid, but I'm no more afraid of this surgery than I am of going to sleep at night. The risk of surgery almost seems obsolete, because if something happens, it's going to happen when I'm asleep. I'm not going to know what hit me, and it'll be over with, it'll be final and my hurting will all be over.' Christie is ready to accept whatever fate offers up. 'If I don't have the surgery I'm going to die, and there's a chance that I will die during surgery, and I'm okay with that too.'

Christie says she knows this might sound selfish, given that she has a five-year-old daughter, but she has started to write a letter explaining everything to Olivia. 'It's so sad because you don't plan on doing this when your child is just beginning her life.' The reality is that Christie is having to worry about her life ending, and she wants to help Olivia understand. There is a very good chance, however, that not only will Christie survive the surgery and make a full recovery, she may well get the life she's always dreamed of. 'I just want to get out. I have dreams of running, and in these dreams I just run and run and run and I don't get tired or out of breath,' she says. Christie dreams of taking Olivia roller-blading and swimming, of going to cinemas with her and being able to fit into the seats. 'More than anything I want to lose weight for my child. Mothers are supposed to be able to do things with their children, to have picnics, to go skating, to run around with them. I can't do any of that. I want so badly to be able to take Olivia on a picnic and sit on the ground with her. I want to be the mother that she needs me to be.'

While Christie is having the operation so she can be a better mother, she is also, she admits, doing it for herself. Christie simply wants to live. 'There are so many little things I want to do that I know most people take for granted, like going to the store or the park, or getting in my car and driving.' Being thin, she says, is a dream she's had since she was five, her daughter's age now. 'I can't wait. I can't wait to be in my new shoes.' When she has lost weight, Christie intends to fulfil another dream. 'I've always wanted to go to Disney World. It was my fantasy and now Olivia has the same dream. Every day she asks, "Can we go to Disney World?" So I've promised her that by the time she turns seven I will take her. I haven't made many promises to her because of my health, but I feel like this one is important. It's kind of subconsciously boosting me up for the future. You know, there is going to be a future,' she smiles. 'I'm going to be in it and Olivia and I are going to be doing everything together.'

Christie Martin's surgery, in March 1998, was a success. By June 1998 she had lost 160lb and she is still losing weight.

The Obesity Surgeon

Every year, Dr George Cowan of the University of Tennessee in Memphis, performs over 300 stomach and intestinal bypass operations on people like Christie. It is his life's work. 'I have a war on obesity. It's a very important war, because this disease killed my father, it killed his mother, my dear nanny, and today it's killing millions of people around the globe. Annually, the loss of life in the United States alone is over 300,000 individuals from obesity and obesity-related diseases.' As part of his crusade, Cowan runs the Obesity Wellness Center at the Baptist Memorial Hospital, where he performs obesity, or bariatric, surgery. He is actually a general surgeon, but over the past 15 years has become increasingly focused on helping the obese. 'It seems to become more and more of a calling for me.' And, he says, there is simply more need for it. 'We have so many large people now, and so many more large people than we've ever had before.' Basically, he says, we are in the midst of a pandemic, a global obesity crisis.

Cowan points out that human beings have evolved over four

million years, and today we have probably the most energy efficient bodies ever. 'At the same time we have a society that is so efficient at reducing our work and energy output, and so we have a collision of these two efficiencies: the efficient human body and the way too energy-efficient modern society. And together,' he says, 'this has produced the disease of obesity.' And with high-calorie, high-fat food so readily available, many people don't stand a chance. 'It's a perfect set up for people in a toxic food environment to be big.' Cowan stresses that genes also play a role in obesity. 'Experts throughout the world agree there is a significant component of genetics and inheritance in obesity,' he says. 'But if you don't have the right genes and the genes are not turned on for obesity, you're not going to be obese.'

However, if you are genetically susceptible to obesity but happen to live somewhere like Bangladesh or Somalia, he says, you are still not going to be big because there is not sufficient food. 'You have to have the appropriate culture, you have to have the appropriate environment with food, plus have the genes and the genes turned on.' To a greater or lesser degree, he says, people inherit the amount of fat that they have. This, he adds, also applies to thin people. 'Thin people can feel satisfied when they've had a certain amount of calories. They can push food away, know when they've had enough and leave food on the plate. It's in their genes,' Cowan believes. What many big people don't seem to have, particularly amongst Cowan's morbidly obese patients, is the ability to feel full. 'Thin people are so fortunate. But so many of them self-righteously puff themselves up and say, "I know when to stop, so why can't they?"'

Discrimination

It is exactly this sort of attitude that so angers Cowan. 'I have a war on obesity because of the gross prejudice, because of the extreme unfairness in our society towards the obese. They're treated as the modern equivalent of lepers, and I'm a leper doctor.' In society we demand that people control themselves, he says. 'Bad people are people who do not conform, and when they do not conform they are punished.' And obese people cannot hide, says Cowan, any more than black people can hide the colour of their skin. 'Obese people are billboards of their own problem.' But today, while racial discrimination is absolutely unacceptable, fat people are seen as fair game. The obese are the last bastion of prejudice. 'There's nothing else, whether it's national origin, religion, race, you name it, the size of your nose, you cannot nail anybody without suffering negative consequences,' he says angrily.

The obese, however, are targets. They are assaulted verbally and physically, or by being totally marginalised and ignored, says Cowan. And people fire arrows into them daily. 'Big people are hit hundreds of times, in one way or another, day after day after day. And they are such bad hits that the obese themselves come to believe falsely that they are bad people, and they start to feel guilty about themselves.' This is fundamentally wrong, he says. 'It's fattism, and it's inhumane and inappropriate for a so-called modern society to allow this to go on.'

Cowan points out that there are so many different reasons people become obese, yet society is largely unsympathetic. 'The obese do not necessarily thumb their nose at society and say, "I'm going to be big". I don't know if anybody's ever tried to get large and stay large. Maybe a Sumo wrestler or two,' he says, 'but certainly not in our culture. Once people get big, they can't lose it. So the blame is not on the individual, but on society for making large people's lives such hell, and for reducing their opportunities for employment and advancement, and for ruining social lives by ignoring or avoiding them.' These are all forms of weight harassment and weight terrorism, he says, and are totally unacceptable. 'America needs to wake up and see what it's doing so unfairly to these individuals. If somebody thinks that they are pure in heart and spirit towards all, yet they dump on fat people by self-right-eously saying, "You just need to push away your plate, zip your lips and you'll lose weight", that's total garbage. People should know better.'

However, Cowan also points out that even those who were once large themselves can sometimes be prejudiced. 'Some who have lost their weight actually enjoy telling big people off, telling them how they can take care of their problem, kind of like reformed smokers,' he says. 'I have a patient who was close to 700 pounds. He'd been housebound for three years, bedbound for a year. He came to me and we dieted him down to a certain point, then I operated on him and he's doing well. He's in about the upper 300 pound range now. But a few months ago when he was with us I went into his room at the hospital and told him about another patient I was going to see, someone who weighed 1,250 pounds. And you know what this man said? He said, "My God, how could he let himself get that way?"'

The Personal Battle

Cowan's crusade stems from a genuine desire to help the obese, and is strengthened by the fact that he watched both his father and grandmother suffer. However, some of his experience is even closer to home. 'Since childhood I've always been a bit chunky. I suspect that having a morbidly obese father and grandmother has some-thing to do with that,' he says. Indeed, his beloved father died weighing 400lb. 'I'm borderline. I'm overweight but not quite obese.' But, he says, he's realistic enough to know he could easily gain more weight. 'So every morning I get on the floor and do about 100 push-ups and 100 sit-ups, and when I get to the hospital I walk up 12 flights of stairs,' he says. This routine has helped to keep his weight in check and build more muscle.

However, Cowan admits to sometimes succumbing to the pull of the fridge. When there's little crunchies and munchies and snacks everywhere, it's hard not to rise to temptation, he says. 'It's so hard when we get a little stressed or a little twang of hunger, not to go and seek those things out. And every one adds a calorie, adds a calorie, adds a calorie. This toxic food environment that we live in is overwhelming if you have a tendency to rise to it. And I rise to it with abandon.'

He admits to sometimes wrestling with himself, going backwards and forwards to the fridge. 'My brain will be saying, "Now George, this is ridiculous. You've got a meal coming up in an hour, you ate not long ago and here you are literally pigging out. What the hell are you doing? You teach this stuff!",' he admits. 'These thoughts flash through my head, but they are actually overcome by another part of my brain which says, "Hey, this stuff is good and you really want some more. Feed me". And it wins. And I go back and I have some more.' Magnify this action and speed up the frame, he says, and what you have is a food bingeing problem. 'I guess I'm more in the middle, and thank God I'm not putting away thousands of calories.' But some people do, and this is partly where the problem lies.

Many of the obese people Cowan treats come to him as a last resort. They have tried every diet, every pill and nothing has worked long-term. 'The fact is that diets don't work.' In the short-term diets can help people to lose weight, but keeping it off, he says, is incredibly difficult. 'It is absurd to think that people are going to be able to take a 1,000 calorie diet for the rest of their lives and stick with it 95 per cent of the time. These things fail.' Dieting, exercise routines and behaviour modification fail within three to five years, he believes. People go back to their old behaviour and therefore end up back at their original weight. 'You have to continue doing the things you need to do, continue with the dieting, the exercise, the appropriate choice of food, and continue with these changes in behaviour,' he says. But completely changing the way you live, and sticking to it, is a very tall order.

In addition, science and medicine still seem to be far away from finding a magic bullet. 'I would love to see medications that are considerably more effective. I'd gladly hang up my scalpel and just go away quietly, but they aren't there at present, and I doubt that it's ever going to be that simple,' he says. Obesity, like cancer or the common cold, is a chronic, continuing human illness which is currently unrelenting in the face of medical therapy. In the light of all this, it is Cowan's firm belief that surgery is at the moment the only thing that works long-term. 'It is not the fault of the individual that they have to come to a surgeon such as myself for bariatric surgery.' Rather it is the failure of medicine to produce anything near to what can be done with surgery.

Obesity Surgery

Dr Cowan performs both gastric (stomach) bypasses and gastrointestinal bypasses, the costs of which are usually covered by medical insurance. The majority of his patients, 70 per cent, are women.

During the stomach bypass, which Cowan calls his 'Memphis bypass', the stomach is divided using stitches and staples, so that a small pouch of about one quarter of the stomach's total size is formed. This essentially blocks off most of the stomach, reducing its functional size to 2 or 3 oz. and leaving the other three quarters unused. As a result, the amount of food that can be eaten, and thus absorbed, is severely limited. Because the stomach becomes so tiny, patients feel full after just a few mouthfuls of food. Sometimes a small ring is also placed around the top part of the pouch, which helps to further restrict patients eating too much or too quickly. When patients need to lose a great deal of weight, Cowan may also perform an intestinal bypass, known at the Roux-en-Y bypass. During this procedure, a section of the colon is removed. This means that the small section of stomach in use now empties directly into the small bowel, bypassing most of the intestines, and so limiting the opportunity for food to be digested and absorbed. Most of Cowan's patients undergo all three procedures.

Most patients lose between 40-50lb. within the first three to four months after surgery. 'By nine months they are down by 100 or more pounds, then it varies after that,' Cowan explains. Some lose half their body weight or more, and most get to within 20lb. of the target weight set before surgery. Studies have shown that the majority of people manage to drop 50 per cent of their weight within a year, and most keep the weight off in the long-term. Studies have also shown that the surgery itself is relatively safe; risk of death during the operation is between one and two per cent. However, complications, such as infection, fistulas and pulmonary problems can occur afterwards, although Cowan stresses these are relatively rare; his complication rate, he says, is a little above five per cent. 'Nationally, the rate for serious complications runs between about five and 10 per cent. But we are dealing with a rather unhealthy segment of the population, and it's amazing that the complication rate is actually that low,' he says.

Cowan points out that while surgery is effective, it is no easy ride, and a solution for only some people. 'It depends how much weight a person needs to lose as to whether surgery is appropriate or not. There are people who are 50 or 60 or 70 pounds overweight, where surgery is not appropriate.' Indeed, a person must be at least 100 pounds overweight before they can be considered. Cowan meets with potential surgery candidates several times, and conducts a number of tests before deciding whether or not to go ahead. Not all morbidly obese patients are necessarily candidates for obesity surgery. 'If someone has a depression which is severe, then it is the wrong time to put added stress on them,' he explains. 'Then there are individuals who may be too heavy for surgery.' These people are so ill that the trauma of surgery could be very dangerous. 'Some people may need to come down by 100 or even 200 pounds before I can operate on them.'

But once the surgery has taken place, the transformation in people is, for Cowan, something of a miracle. 'This surgery is unique. We're taking people where they've never been before,' he says. Indeed, 68 per cent of Cowan's patients have been big since they were children; they have never known what it is like to have a thin body. 'This is exciting, because you're helping people whose quality of life has been poor.' Barely being able to get through the day, he says, is no way to live. 'But then they lose their weight, perhaps 30, even 50 per cent of their weight, and suddenly they're full of energy. They take a second job or go back to school; they get promotions, they get a mate if they don't already have one. And life is so beautiful and so incredibly positive.' These are people who have always been outcasts, avoided like the plague, he points out. 'And now they are going where they've never been before,' he smiles. For Cowan, it is a wonderful gift he is able to give people. 'It's very satisfying and gratifying.'

And while Cowan wants the best for all his patients, ultimately, he acknowledges, it is up to the individual. 'I'm here to help people, but I'm not here as a policeman to tell them, "You will do this". My role is more to guide them as a friend.' Many patients are marvellous and very motivated, and do very well, he says. 'I wish everyone could be like that, but we work with humanity, and a wide breadth of it.' Some people, he explains, do respond in self-destructive ways, and some even manage to outfox their surgery. 'There are people who eat through their surgery, by drinking liquid chocolate, colas, liquid ice-cream.' These cases, however, are rare. Experience has taught Cowan the best way to help and encourage people during the difficult times following surgery. 'I've found the most effective way to help people is simply to love them and care for them,' he smiles.

Surgery: The Reality

Lisa Pike is the Nurse Manager at Dr Cowan's Obesity Wellness
Center. She has helped hundreds of patients through obesity
surgery, and knows only too well what the reality is. 'It's no picnic
at all,' she stresses. 'The surgery is a major lifestyle change.
Basically, everything in the patient's life changes, and it's not something you can do by yourself. People need a lot of support and
encouragement to adjust.'

Food

The most drastic change for patients to cope with is the fact they
can only eat up to three ounces of food at a time. 'One day you're
having a steak and baked potato, and suddenly the next day after
surgery, you'll probably never have a meal of that size again.' After
the operation, patients need to eat five or six meals each day, either
in liquid form or pureed; many eat baby food. Once they adjust to
this new way of life, they can progress onto solid food and may be
able to eat three meals a day, though still only very small portions.
'We give patients a special restaurant card which says, "Please give
this person a child's portion". That way they don't have to pay for
a full portion they'll never be able to eat,' explains Lisa. If patients
do eat too much and over-fill their pouch, the body reacts instantly:
they will vomit.

Vitamins

The surgery may cause malabsorption of some nutrients, so
patients need to have their vitamin and electrolyte levels checked
every three months initially, then every six months and finally every
year, for life. 'They may get a vitamin D or calcium deficiency, for
example, and it's important they comply with the regimen and take
a lot of pills and medicines,' says Lisa.

Toilet

Because the operation causes food to pass straight through patients, they have bowel movements much more frequently. 'You go to the bathroom sometimes eight or nine times a day,' says Lisa. 'It can seem like every time you turn round mum's in the bathroom, or your wife's in the bathroom. And,' she adds, 'people have a lot of gas and a lot of belching, and that can be unattractive. It has actually turned a lot of spouses off, and people have had relationship problems just because of this.'

Relationships

The extreme weight loss caused by surgery can also cause difficulties in relationships. 'The weight loss is hard for a lot of people to handle,' explains Lisa. 'As the woman or man loses weight they become more attractive. Women notice guys are looking at them, sometimes for the first time in their lives, and spouses can become jealous. You can actually have serious relationship problems, even divorce, as a result of dramatic weight loss.'

George's Angels

Because people need so much assistance after surgery, Dr Cowan set up a support group called George's Angels. Run by patients, the group organises get-togethers and keeps people in touch via regular newsletters. There are currently 1,500 members.

Words Of Warning

'The surgical procedures for obesity are only relevant for a small minority of people,' cautions Professor Kelly Brownell of Yale University. 'Only a small fraction of people are overweight enough to justify the risks of surgery. But for people who are massively overweight and have a seriously increased health risk, surgery can be life saving in some cases.' For people with 100 or 200 or more pounds to lose, he says, the thought of doing it gradually by making lifestyle changes is daunting indeed. 'Some people can do that, but not many. The question then becomes, "What do you do to help such people?" and surgery can be really helpful.'

However, the fact that there is even a need for obesity surgery angers Brownell. 'Just as it makes me angry that we have to have treatments for emphysema when people smoke, because emphysema doesn't have to occur, and we don't have to have cigarettes.' In the same way, he says, we don't have to have obesity; if we didn't have such a bad food environment, we wouldn't have so many obese people. 'But the fact is that we do have these things, and something needs to be done.' Surgery does have a place. 'But it's a sad statement that somebody has to deform their body, has to take an otherwise healthy organ like their stomach and have surgery performed on it in order to remedy this problem.'

'I am a candidate for weight-loss surgery. I think my BMI is 45. But when I go to those bariatric surgery conferences, I feel I am walking into a den of people who look at me and want to carve me up,' says Marilyn Wann, editor of *Fat?So!* magazine and member of NAAFA, the US National Association to Advance Fat Acceptance. 'For a stomach surgeon to say he's fighting discrimination by carving fat people down to size is insane to me. Those doctors are making money, they are not fighting discrimination. This may be a crude analogy, but it's as though they were taking black people and dropping them into baths of acid to turn them white, then claiming they are helping them avoid discrimination.'

Dr Cowan says he absolutely sympathises with fat acceptance groups' calls to end discrimination against the overweight. 'I'm in complete accord and sympathy with NAAFA,' he says, except with regard to their opinion of surgery. 'I believe their protest is largely related to denial, and denial is a very deep, very wide and very vicious river. I think these people are telling themselves, "I'm fine, I can live this happy life even though I'm big".' But this, he says, is avoiding the obvious. 'As they become more disabled, they have more problems, their quality of life is intruded upon and their lives are shortened,' he says. 'And if they say otherwise, I think they're kidding themselves.'

Lynn McAfee of the US Council on Size and Weight Discrimination is a 500lb. 'fat activist' who has battled with her weight, and prejudice, her whole life. She has in the past considered obesity surgery, but has come to believe it is barbaric. 'I have an open mind about pills, but I do not have an open mind about stomach stapling. I have seen too many people harmed by it. I have had too many calls in the middle of the night from people who say they wish they were dead, people who can't go out any more because they throw up too often and have too much diahorrea, people who have lost most of their hair,' she says. 'Stomach stapling is a barbaric practice and it's based on misinformation about size; it is based on the premise that obese people all eat enormous amounts of food every day.' Many obese people, she says, do not eat more than the average sized person and yet are still fat. 'The surgery is based on a very old and very inexact science, and people get very sick after this operation.'

Becky Smith: Life After Surgery

'Before the operation I weighed 340 pounds, and I looked pitiful. I was 64 and a half inches in the waist, my arms were big, my face was big and it was just a nightmare. I could barely walk, I could barely breathe, and the only enjoyment I got out of life was food. I felt very ugly and just didn't feel like I belonged. I gave a great show when I was out, pretending I was happy, but I would get home and die on the inside because I was so miserable and unhappy. It was just a horrible life. I look back now and I cannot believe that was me.

'I've really tried to figure out why I got so big, and I think when it comes down to it, it's basically food. But you have to figure out what problems you have in your life and solve them, in order to understand your food problems. I had a really hard childhood. I had a lot of trauma in my childhood, things that people don't know about, things I had to deal with myself, and I think I just turned to food for comfort. I had to conquer those things, and it was really tough. I always looked pretty good growing up, and sometimes people looked at me and said things in the wrong way, and I would always blame myself because of the way I looked. So I think gaining weight was a shield, so that no one would look at me like that or say ugly things to me.

'With food, I could not control myself. Sometimes if I couldn't decide what I wanted for lunch, I would go to four different fast food places, get meals from all of them, and take them home and eat them all. And that's when I was at my happiest. Or if I went to a drive-through hamburger place, I would get three hamburgers, three orders of fries, three desserts and three large cokes so that the people in the restaurant would think I was getting food for three different people. I looked to food for everything. When I was sad it would comfort me. When I was tired or lonely, it was always there for me. When nobody else was, or nothing else was, food was there, and it made me feel good.

'But I got to the point where I couldn't breathe and I couldn't walk. Years ago I'd wanted to lose weight so I'd look good. I would hear older people say, "I just want to do it for my health" and I didn't know what they were talking about. But at 43 years old, I started thinking about my health. I couldn't live like that any more, and so I decided to have surgery. I told all my friends that if I were to die during the operation, to know I was resting in peace, that nobody would ever make fun of me again, that I'd never be fat and miserable again. But, if I got through surgery, the same would apply; I would lose weight and nobody would make fun of me again and I would be happy. I wanted so badly to be normal. The whole time they were wheeling me down to the operating room I just cried. I was rejoicing one minute then petrified the next. But I was prepared for whatever God dealt out for me. I'd reached the point where I was afraid to live, but I was no longer afraid to die.

'As far as I'm concerned, my birthday is May 3rd, 1996, the day I had my operation. I am a new person now, but it's funny because I don't really know who this person is; I'm getting to know myself again. But at last I'm normal. I can go to a restaurant and sit anywhere. When I go to the theatre I don't have to sit in the handicapped section. When I sit in a chair I don't have to push my fat in on the sides. When I go to a buffet, people aren't snickering at me for getting food. People even go out of their way to open doors for me now. But sometimes I get mad at these men I've never met before who open doors for me, because I wonder if they would have done that two years ago.

'After the operation, when you lose an extreme amount of weight, your skin can sag. My stomach hung pretty low and I got a hernia. There was also an irritated area where the skin hung over and got blistered and rubbed red and raw, so I had a tummy tuck. They pulled my waistline in 3 inches and took 8 to 10 pounds of fat off my stomach. I also chose to have a breast reduction, because it's all just fat; breasts get fat like everything else. I've chosen not to have my arms or legs done, but that's there too if I want it.

'Now I also know what it's like to feel full. Everybody else knows what it's like to feel full or leave a piece of bread or meat or vegetable on your plate. But when you're morbidly obese, if you're sitting at a table with 10 people, nobody sends food back. The morbidly obese person is going to eat everything on everybody's plate. We just have to eat it all. And now I am like everybody else. I get full, I eat smaller amounts and when I'm full, I push back whatever's left on the plate. But it's true this surgery is a commitment. You need to take vitamins and make sure you have enough protein and you really need to think about what you're going to eat for the day. The thing about surgery is that you eat many more meals, you eat smaller amounts several times a day, but that's kind of fun too.

'I'm so happy now, but there is another side of me that gets really angry. I was at a dance club one night and I was standing next to two or three gentlemen, and they were trying to talk to me and my friend. We were all watching some girls dance. They were quite heavy, but they were out there dancing and they were dancing better than anybody else. Then one of the men leaned over and said to me, "Isn't that disgusting. Look at those pigs out there trying to dance". I said, "Wait right here", and I went out to my car and got a picture, and came back and said to him, "This is what I looked like a year and a half ago, and I don't appreciate you saying that. Those women there are people just like you and me. They're good people. Don't ever talk about fat people like that". And he was shocked and very apologetic and said he'd learned something.

'Now I spread the word to others, that's my gift. Dr Cowan gave me a gift, and I give it back whenever I get the chance. If there's a morbidly obese person standing behind me in the grocery line, I'll reach over and grab a candy bar and say, "I think I'm going to get this. I deserve it. I've lost 212 pounds'. Well, the obese person will immediately ask me how I did it. I just say, "Here's my name and number, this is what I've done, it's been great. Call me if you're interested". But one thing I will never do is try to talk anybody into surgery. They have to decide for themselves. I just show them how it has benefited me and a hundred other people I know. So yes, I will go out of my way. I've done it many times, and I will probably do it five or six times today. I believe obesity is a disease, and what I tell people is that if a blind man had a chance to see, he would take it. I had my own chance to see, and I took it.'

CHAPTER EIGHT

THE BEAUTY OF FAT: BIG, POSITIVE WOMEN

Melanie Coles

'I wake up every morning and think, "Right, what can I do today to make a change?"'

Melanie Coles is a 26-year-old London-based photographer with a mission. Through her work she is striving to help big women develop the self-esteem and self-respect so often denied them by society. 'I focus on big women because I am one, and because I feel that we've never had the level of self-respect that is our right and that we deserve.' Some women, she says, have never even experienced positive images of themselves. 'I try to make images that prove they are beautiful and worthy. I try to give them back what has been stolen.'

Melanie has always been big. 'I think I'm this shape because I was born this way. Most of it is down to genetics. Everyone in my family is big, my sister, my mother, my grandmother, and my aunties.' And although at times she struggles with it, Melanie is learning to be at home with her body. 'I feel fit. I can run for a bus. I go to water aerobics once or twice a week, I swim as much as I can and I walk everywhere.' Some of her friends, Melanie points out, are thin but definitely not fit. 'They smoke like chimneys, eat terribly and drink lots of alcohol. I eat good food, and I make an effort because I want to be healthy. And just because I have excess flesh,' she says, 'doesn't make me any less fit.'

But having excess flesh does affect Melanie in other ways. 'I feel excluded a lot of the time, whether it's shopping or just sitting in a restaurant,' she admits. 'I'll walk down the street and see an advertising image of a beautiful girl in a beautiful dress, and I'm reminded that that's not available to me. There are about three shops on the average high street that I can possibly go into, and hundreds of others that I can't.' And this can be humiliating. 'I might want the beautiful dress my girlfriend is wearing but I can never find it. Clothes start at size 8 and it's boom, boom, boom, finished at 16. It's as though I don't exist. If I'm not within that bracket, the message is, "Get out".' Instead, Melanie, who is a size 20, has a collection of handbags, jewellery and shoes to rival Imelda Marcos. 'I have to resort to a huge shoe collection and bags galore, and it's funny and I'm famous for them among my friends.' But, she says, it is also quite sad. 'It's a reminder that I don't fit in. It's as simple as that.'

And reminders of this come in many forms. 'I was recently on a packed bus in the middle of Oxford Street and I had two heavy shopping bags with me. I accidentally knocked this girl with one of the bags, and immediately went to apologise.' But Melanie wasn't given the chance. 'She just looked at me and said, "Jesus Christ you're fat. Look at you, you don't deserve to be on this bus." She was screaming at me because I'd annoyed her, and she thought she had the right to humiliate me. She went on and on and on, and I just wanted to dig a hole in the bus and through Oxford Street and all the way home.' Melanie was so shocked she was lost for words. 'I just couldn't think of a clever answer for her.'

Melanie believes incidents like this may be the unpleasant result of fear and lack of understanding. 'Perhaps people don't realise that you can be fat *and* happy and healthy. They think, "How can you walk down the street and have a smile on your face. It's not your right". It confuses them because it's not the general view.' Fear and negativity, it seems, are woven into the very fabric of society. 'I open magazines and see beautiful clothes on girls who are not just thin, they're super-tiny. I switch on the television and see Richard and Judy's one millionth attempt to get the nation to be something we can't all be, or

I hear on the Nine O'clock News that there's some new diet pill.' Added to this, she says, the medical profession constantly sends out the message that being overweight is dangerous and unhealthy.

'I read articles that tell me, "If you're overweight you're going to get this disease and that disease, blah, blah, blah",' she says. 'That hurts, because it's not necessarily true. It's just a constant kick in the teeth, and I can't escape it because it's everywhere.' And everywhere the message is that we must strive for perfection. 'You have to be a certain type of person. You have to be a mother, a career woman, a socialite. You have to be intelligent and beautiful and wear the right clothes. You have to have the right job, the right car, the right home and the right child.' And you have to be thin.

And as a result, the fear of fat just grows stronger. 'I see the looks people give me and my family, I hear the little jibes,' says Melanie. 'Throughout my life I've been bombarded with negative messages about being big, and so has everyone else.' And everyone fears getting fat. 'It's frightening for people. No one wants to put on a couple of stones, or even a couple of pounds.' Through talking to friends of different shapes and sizes, Melanie has come to realise that everybody is insecure. 'People are constantly talking about what they ate, what they didn't eat, how many sit-ups they did last night. Friends who might be a fraction of my size will talk about how big their thighs or arms are, and I'll think, "Hang on a minute, what does that say about me? What does that mean I am?"' And even if Melanie's having a good day and feeling good about herself, she can't escape it. 'It's always there, worming and grinding away.'

But she never stops fighting to maintain her sense of self. 'I wake up every morning and think, "Right, what can I do today to make a change?" Every day I fight against it. I'd definitely call myself an activist. I want change. I want things to be better, and I believe very strongly they should be better. We should be equal and we should have the same opportunities as everyone else.' And as someone who is dedicated to creating beautiful images of large people, Melanie feels particularly responsible.

'There is a need, a hunger for more positive images of women.' And with an estimated 47 per cent of women size 16 or over, this is not surprising. 'Statistically, we deserve our proportion. We deserve images to be out there for us, and for everybody else, to prove we can be fit, and we can be happy, healthy and sexy. We can be all those things. Just let us get on with it.' And people need to be educated to celebrate and accept differences, Melanie says. 'We're not all the same weight, the same colour or the same sex. Size is just another difference, it's part of who you are as an individual.' And images we see everywhere should simply include larger people. 'Things need to be opened up. There's some fantastic big women and girls out there. Use them.'

Melanie did just this when she recently worked on a groundbreaking campaign for The Body Shop, called Love Your Body. 'I took photographs of a plus-size model called Beatrice Appleby for a poster campaign. It was a huge celebration of empowerment; Beatrice was just so empowered by her body, by her sheer beauty. She's so full of life,' Melanie smiles. 'The whole idea was to prove that you can be big and beautiful.' The finished image showed Beatrice bursting though lots of bubbles, laughing happily. 'Love Your Body is exactly the right message, and I know it made a difference to some people. If I can produce images that change even one person's life, then that's one person more than yesterday.' Melanie says working on the campaign was personally life-changing. 'And it helped my family too. They loved it, and whenever I've spoken about it or watched people's reactions in the shop, the response has been really positive.'

Despite the difficulties and the anger she often feels, Melanie's sense of who she is and where she belongs grows stronger and stronger. 'I would say I'm big and happy. I try to get on with my life and not let anything stop me. Most days, if I'm surrounded by people who love me, who know and respect me, then I can get up in the morning with a smile on my face and do something positive. I think that's important.'

Jackqueline Hope

'I love having large breasts, I love having big hips and a little belly. To me, I'm Rubenesque. I look in the mirror and I like what I see. And who the hell is out there to tell me that anything is wrong with it?'

Jackqueline Hope weighs over 200lb. She is often described as curvaceous and voluptuous and, until recent times, would have been widely considered not only fashionable, but a desirable icon. 'For a very long time the full figure was idealised,' she says. 'If women had big busts, and big hips and thighs they were thought of as the cream of the crop, as being strong and wealthy. And we know that for a long time men enjoyed bigger busts and bigger hips.' Once, having a large woman on your arm was a sign of success. 'Today it has completely changed. It is now almost a disgrace for men to be seen with large women, although I honestly believe a lot of men do like larger women, they're just so afraid of how society will perceive them.' Unfortunately, all hell broke loose after the Twiggy look evolved in the 1960s, says Jackqueline. This was when the media, and the world, began to idealise the thin body. 'And a lot of people who were bigger than Twiggy felt they had to lose weight. That's when the revolution started.'

Since then, society has deemed it necessary to look a specific way in order to be accepted, Jackqueline says. 'If someone is larger you feel they're unkempt and unsuccessful, that they're dirty and lack willpower. And it's so untrue.' Indeed, the world large-sized people inhabit is very scary, she says. But while Jackqueline believes the media is partly to blame for all of this, she also feels people must take responsibility for themselves. 'I truly believe it's a result of individuals not believing in themselves and not liking who they are. I think it comes from within.' The problem is, we allow ourselves to get caught up in this perception of the ideal. 'We blame ourselves because we don't look like the person next door, or the person on the magazine cover. We think we're not good enough and that we don't measure up,' she says. 'I think we have to love ourselves as individuals, and really appreciate ourselves for the way that we are. I mean, God made chihuahuas and he made great danes, and I look at myself as being a great dane in life.'

While in her 20s, Jackqueline became Canada's first plus-size model, and in 1981 founded a company called Big, Bold & Beautiful. Today, that business includes Canada's largest plus-size modelling agency as well as two Toronto-based clothing boutiques, Big, Bold & Beautiful and Big, Bold & Beautiful Brides. Jackqueline also designs plus-size clothes for her shops, and gets special pleasure from helping larger brides-to-be find their ideal wedding gown. Having gone down the aisle twice herself, she understands the difficulty. 'A woman is supposed to be a princess on her wedding day,' she says. However, for a large woman who may never have been the centre of attention before, the whole experience can be frightening. 'I try to give brides the self-esteem and confidence they need to go down the aisle. I tell them they're truly, uniquely beautiful at the size they are.'

To get to this point, however, Jackqueline has had to make her own, often difficult, journey. 'I was in despair for a long time,' she admits. 'At my heaviest I weighed 340 pounds. I loved food, it was my comfort, my joy, my friend to go home to at night when I was feeling depressed and lonely. Yet it became my enemy when I wanted to be something other than what I was,' she says. 'For a very long time I was on a constant merry-go-round, trying to get to a size society would perceive as acceptable.' For a while she binged and purged, and became anorexic. 'It was a vicious circle.' Like so many other women, Jackqueline also tried lots of diets and became depressed if she didn't lose weight. 'I felt very unsuccessful, so I would turn to food again. The sad thing is that I didn't really have control over my life. Food had the control. It was in the driver's seat and I was just going along for the ride. That was a very frightening experience.'

While going from diet clinic to diet clinic, Jackqueline met a woman called Darlene who weighed over 500lb. 'She was a wonderful woman. She didn't have a lot of friends, but to me she was beautiful. She was fun to be with, she laughed out loud, she had a joy and a love that to this day I have never found in anyone.' Despite this, Darlene's husband wanted her to lose weight. 'We were both there to lose weight, and both there because our husbands wanted us to be.' One day the friends went for their regular weigh-in at a clinic, and to their delight found they had both lost weight. 'We decided to go and celebrate by having a lovely donut and a cup of coffee,' Jackqueline remembers. 'As we were going to the elevator I realised I had forgotten my allotment of shakes for the week, and I told Darlene I would catch up with her in the lobby.'

Five minutes later, Jacqueline returned to find her friend lying on the floor. She had died from a heart attack. 'I saw the ambulance drivers coming towards her, making fun of her weight saying, "We've got a big one here. We'll need help lifting her onto a stretcher".' At that moment, Jackqueline realised she didn't even know Darlene's last name, but it didn't matter. 'I'd known her from the inside. She was an angel and angels don't have last names.' Her friend's death was the beginning of an enormous change in outlook for Jackqueline. In fact, it was in Darlene's memory that she started Big, Bold & Beautiful. 'I started the company because I didn't want other people to go on 500-calorie-a-day diets, trying to become the thin person somebody else wanted them to be.'

Another catalyst for change was Jackqueline's uneasy relationship with the medical profession. 'For many years I was extraordinarily frightened of going to the doctor. It got to the point where every time I went, even with a common case of 'flu, it would end in a lecture about my weight,' she explains. When she wasn't feeling very good about herself in the first place, these experiences were traumatic. 'So I stopped going.' Three years later, when she finally had to go because she felt so ill, Jackqueline was diagnosed as having diabetes. 'I was told that there was no choice but for me to be put on insulin.' Frightened, and realising how important her health was to her, Jackqueline decided to adopt a healthier and more active lifestyle. 'And I lost over 160 pounds,' she says, 'but I look at that simply as a side-effect of getting very healthy.' She now wishes she'd been able to go to the doctor much earlier, and saved herself years of feeling unwell. 'But because I was so frightened, I ignored that.'

Jackqueline is very concerned that doctors too often make blanket judgements, and unnecessarily scare so many people. 'I think the medical profession must loosen up a little bit. It's very difficult to be told time after time that if you don't fit within their realms of healthy weight, you're not healthy. Whoever made up those weight charts is absolutely ridiculous,' she states. What matters is whether people who are large are also healthy, she says. Unfortunately, the reality is that patients are randomly told to lose weight.

'I think the medical profession has a lot to do with people getting stuck in the yo-yo dieting cycle.' And too many people, she says, go through years of unnecessary despair. 'There's an awful lot of people who are worrying about their weight for purely aesthetic reasons. I think if you're trying to look like Cindy Crawford, you should forget about it,' she says. 'If you're healthy but don't happen to look like that, you have to just get on with your life and enjoy every single minute.'

However, if someone is unhealthy, as Jackqueline herself was, it's time to act. 'Then you must start moving and get active and listen to your doctor,' she says. And some people may need to lose weight. 'I do believe there's an extreme as far as weight goes. There's a lot of people out there who are very obese and very unhappy and unhealthy. There are people who can't walk or who are bedridden, and they are probably very frightened, addicted to food and trapped in a lifestyle they can't escape from. That's when something has to be done.'

Jackqueline believes it's people at this extreme that the medical profession really should address, rather than placing all overweight people in the 'danger' category. 'It's very difficult for people such as myself, who may be 20, 40, or 50 pounds overweight, because we feel bulked in with those who are 500 pounds overweight.' However, she adds, some people do go to the other extreme and lose too much weight. 'They don't know when to stop because there's no borderline. I have very thin girlfriends who are about 120 pounds, yet feel they're 20 pounds overweight.'

Anxiety, Jackqueline says, is often at the root of these problems. 'I think we need to realise that beauty comes in all shapes and sizes.' Worry simply makes people struggle to be something they were never meant to be. 'I cannot see myself as a size 8. That's a whole other world. To me, being a size 8 is the impossible nightmare, never mind the impossible dream.' And forget about the notion that losing weight will solve all your problems, she says. 'What you've got to do is take every single moment and live it to the fullest, because you might not be around tomorrow.' This realisation was Jackqueline's turning point. 'When I knew I had diabetes and there was a possibility I might die, I started to look at life as being very precious,' she says. And it had nothing to do with needing to be 20lb. lighter. 'It was living now with the body I had.'

And no matter how hard it feels, she stresses, we can all change our lives. 'I gained control by finally looking at what I was doing to myself and realising that I was the only one who had control over my hand going to my mouth. If I wanted to live, and love food and be happy, I had to take control.' She still loves food, but in a different way. 'Now *I* have control over *it*.' Exercise has also become an integral part of Jackqueline's every day life. 'I am extraordinarily healthy. If I was challenged by a 120 pound person who does not work out, I could beat them 10 times over. I weigh over 200 pounds, but I work out for two hours, five days a week and there's nothing wrong with me.'

As a result of this new outlook, Jackqueline's life has changed in every way. 'Now I have a full length mirror and I can stand naked and vulnerable in front of it, and look at myself. I can love my hills and valleys and my dimples and imperfections; I can love every single inch because I know it has a history. I know that my body has been through an awful lot and it's been good to me in times of trouble. My body has strength and warmth and personality, and I really have to celebrate that.' And this includes celebrating her own sexuality. 'Big people don't talk about having sex. Big people are not supposed to be sexy. They're not supposed to walk into the bedroom with the lights on and throw themselves at their lover,' she says. 'For many years of my life, particularly in my first marriage, I wasn't seen as an attractive woman. I lived the life of a woman who wasn't supposed to show her sensuality, or bare her soul or feel anything intimate.'

But once she started loving herself and her body, Jackqueline's sensual side emerged. 'There were days when I would do my housekeeping in the nude, and dance with the broom to soft music and candlelight. I would sing along to Joe Cocker's 'You're So Beautiful To Me', and believe in myself and love myself.' In her book, *Big, Bold and Beautiful*, Jackqueline includes a chapter on sexuality. 'It was hard to write, but I wanted people to know they can have fun in the bedroom, they can enjoy their heavier thighs and their protruding tummies, their swaying breasts and big hips. And they can make their lover enjoy it all too, without any inhibitions,' she smiles.

However, she acknowledges, getting to this stage can be difficult. 'For many years I felt no warmth as a large-sized woman. I felt that no one wanted to touch me, that they thought I was contagious. I had so much love bottled up inside me for so long and no one to reach out and touch, no one to share it with,' Jackqueline says. With Big, Bold & Beautiful, however, she has created a place large women can go to feel accepted and celebrated just as they are. 'A lot of people do not give you that chance. They look at the exterior and think, "It's not necessary to talk to her. She's a second-class citizen". Although many of us are larger than life, we're the first to be ignored.' That, she says, has always blown her mind. 'Reach out and touch us. We're living, breathing people in here, we've got hearts the size of Mount Everest, and souls as big as you can get,' she says. 'Through my company I reach out and love as many people as possible. I want to touch them, and I want them to know they're not repulsive.' Her dream is to lead people to the land of the guilt-free. 'I was allowed to go there, and it's a most beautiful land when you allow yourself into it.'

Jackqueline is now exactly as she wants to be. She has a loving and devoted husband and son, and wouldn't have things any other way. 'I work out with a trainer now and I say, "I don't want to lose any more weight. Make me firm and build me up. Make me look fabulous at the weight I am." I like food,' she continues, 'and I refuse to stop eating to be an anorexic-looking woman. I refuse to stop eating to make other people satisfied with the weight they think I should be. I like being a big woman. I love having large breasts, I love having big hips and a little belly. To me, I'm Rubenesque. I look in the mirror and I like what I see. And who the hell is out there to tell me that anything is wrong with it?' she asks. 'I don't want to be Cindy Crawford. I like being Jackqueline Hope.'

Christine Alt

'I started plus-size modelling 12 years ago, and I've worked so much more than I ever did as a straight size model... Having been in both ends of the modelling industry, I want people to know that beauty really knows no size.'

'I started modelling straight out of high school. I was about a size 10/12, and modelling agencies in New York told me I needed to lose weight. I joined an agency and tried every diet there was; the grapefruit diet, the hard-boiled egg diet, this diet, that diet. I even tried chewing but not swallowing, which was my favourite, but I never really lost weight. Then I signed with another agency and got serious. I started going to a nutritionist who helped me lose my first 10 pounds. Then I noticed that if ate less food and exercised more I could lose a lot more weight, and that's how the whole roller coaster started. I ate less and less and exercised for up to three hours a day, and eventually I got down to a size 4. I remember going to get weighed at my agency, and they said, "You're doing great on your diet. Keep it up". I took that to mean lose more weight. I weighed about 110 pounds.

'The industry is obsessed with ultra-thinness. They were trying to groom me for the collections in Milan, and that meant having to be hanger thin, a clothes hanger. The industry really demands that you make your body a size it's not supposed to be. When I hear modelling agency owners say their models aren't anorexic or bulimic, I find it very hard to believe that the thousands and thousands of models in the United States are all naturally a size 6. It's not true.

'I decided, after three years of being ultra-thin in the modelling profession, that I'd had enough. I really had no life, and I realised life was too short to starve myself and spend all my time working out. Somebody once said to me they thought I was obnoxious and stuck up because I wouldn't go out to dinner with them. What they didn't understand is that I *couldn't* go out to dinner because then I would be tempted to eat. Something in me finally woke up, and I walked away from modelling.

'When I started living a normal life, my weight naturally went up to about a size 16, and now I have levelled out to a 14. I definitely think that's the natural weight for my body to be. I think everyone has a natural weight, and for some it's heavier than others. I also truly believe that if I'd never gone down to a size 4, I would probably still be the size I was in high school. I think I hurt myself by losing that much weight and ended up bigger than I should have been. But my body's comfortable where it is now. I eat healthily and I don't restrict myself if I have a craving. I believe in moderation.

'When I stopped modelling I began working as a personal assistant for my sister, the model Carol Alt. One day we were at a modelling convention, and someone approached me and asked me to be a plus-size model. That was a very happy day in my life, because it meant I could finally do something I loved, but without having to nearly kill myself to do it. I started plus-size modelling 12 years ago, and I've worked so much more than I ever did as a straight size model.

'Unfortunately, though, we tend to idolize thinness. There's that old saying, "You can never be too thin or too rich". We put rich people on a pedestal and think of them as icons, and we do the same with thin people. A lot of designers design specifically for thin women; magazines also promote the idea of thinness. Then our young children see these things and think, "This is what I have to look like in order to achieve any form of success". I also think people associate being healthy with being thin, which to me is the biggest fallacy of all. When I was a size 4, I was so much sicker than I've ever been at size 14. I think, as a society, we have to change our vision of what success is and what health is. Being ultra-thin is not healthy.

'And I think there's nothing more ridiculous than turning on the television and seeing an advertisement for a weight loss centre, followed by an advertisement for a fast-food chain. In my neighbourhood there is a block that has an ice-cream store at one end, a donut store at the other, and a weight loss centre right in the middle. I think that's just hysterical, and it's the perfect example of what our society has become.

'But that's only part of it. I think a main problem is that we're all so busy. We put so much emphasis on career and working that we don't have time to go home and cook a meal. So what happens? We go to McDonald's or Burger King and eat that type of food instead of sitting at home and having a nice salad or chicken breast or something. As a society we have to learn how to eat better. We need a variety of different foods and we have to find a good balance. Then we probably wouldn't need all the diets and the diet industry.

'We also have to do some form of exercise to maintain health, but without being fanatical about it. You can exercise and you can have a hamburger, but you have to do it in moderation. We forget that we don't have to listen to the advertising agencies, and that we should find a balance that's good for us. Listen to your inner self. Listen to your heart, to what you know is right for you. I believe everything in moderation, including moderation.

'And you know, it's interesting the tributes women get when they have a little bit more weight on them. I got asked out on a lot more dates, but it was also interesting to get a female point of view. Female friends came up to me and said, "When you were so thin you seemed dead, you had no life in your eyes. Now you're beautiful, you have so much more life and you're a much more pleasurable person to be around". So from both male and female perspectives, I'm more attractive at a larger size than when I was very thin.

'Having been in both ends of the modelling industry, I want people to know that beauty really knows no size. You do not have to be a perfect size 6 or size 8 to be beautiful. I want women to know that just because you're not this perfect size the advertising industry says you should be, it doesn't mean you're less of a woman. You are still beautiful, you are still sexy, and you are still a woman.'

Dawn French

'When I'm thinner, I'm not sure how to be. I'm less comfortable when I don't have the body that fits me.'

'I've often asked myself why I've got the confidence I've got, and I think it has something to do with my childhood. I don't remember any cruelty at all. I was brought up in a very positive, nurturing family who never made my weight an issue.' In fact, she says, it was quite the opposite. 'I think I owe a lot of my innate confidence to my father. He knew he had to make sure my self-esteem was buoyed up and that he had to protect me from those who might decide to reduce my confidence.'

Dawn remembers one particular night as a teenager when she was about to go out to a club. 'I was very nervous about it, and my father knew I was going with a lot of thin girlfriends, and that there was the potential there for cruelty,' she explains. 'He called me into a room and sat me down, and I was ready to get in a huff because I thought I was going to hear the usual litany about not drinking too much and what time I had to be in, and not to get too involved with boys.'

Instead, her father completely surprised her. 'He did something I've never forgotten. He went into this kind of great overture of praise for me. He told me, very calmly, that I was completely beautiful, that I should be proud of myself physically and that of course I was going to be desirable to all the boys I would meet that night. In fact, I was probably going to be the most desirable girl out of all my friends, and therefore, being such a fantastically attractive woman, I was going to have to be on my guard. But he said any boy who managed to get a bit of a snog with me was lucky, and that I should never devalue myself.

'Well, my chest just got bigger and bigger and bigger the more he spoke. And it was very clever, because of course he succeeded in making me so proud of myself, and making my self-esteem so very high, that I wasn't going to let any boy kiss me at all that night. I was just too good,' she laughs. This was simply the most fantastic gift a father could give to his daughter. 'In fact it's always stayed with me, because I believed he was right and I still believe he's right.'

However, Dawn knows that allowing yourself to be big in this world can be difficult. 'I think you have to be pretty strong to remain big, if you are naturally big, which my family is.' Especially given the constant references to some ideal most people can never fit. 'And which doesn't reflect anything that you are.' Dawn admits, however, to falling for the image of the thin ideal on one occasion. 'When I got married I didn't think it was possible to be fat and wear a white dress. I'd never seen a single image that reflected that as an okay thing. I was weak and I regret it,' she says. She didn't want to be a fat bride, so Dawn did something many, many others have done.

'I went to a quack who gave me amphetamines and a shot in the bum, and I paid a lot of money.' The doctor also recommended a diet consisting solely of meat and citrus fruit. 'I smelt repulsive, like an old cadaver, and I was ravenous the whole time. But the pounds just dropped off.' They would, she says, because her body was in such trauma. 'It's kind of eating itself, trying to get any nutrients it can. But yes, I went from a size 24 to a size 10-12 for my wedding day, and I felt very odd. I just didn't know how to use that body and I don't know who I was on that day.' Added to that, she was so ravenous she could hardly wait to get to the reception and eat. 'I was so preoccupied by the thought of food that I couldn't think of anything else.'

Dieting, Dawn says, took her body to a place it didn't belong. 'When I'm thinner, I'm not sure how to be. I'm less comfortable when I don't have the body that fits me, which is the body I have now.' This is the weight she instinctively feels is right. 'We're all short and wide in my family, so it's pointless to battle against that.

I've got no desire to, and in fact I find comfort in it, knowing I belong to this family because I'm this shape.' Her weight does go up and down a bit, she says. 'It depends on what I'm doing, and how active I'm being.'

But Dawn can always tell if she needs to lose a bit of weight. 'I get clues. I know if I'm a bit breathless, or I can't dance for half an hour, or swim or do my job. If I can't be in a play every night because I'm too tired, I know these things are possibly weight-related, and I have the ability to lose a few pounds if I need to.' But it's never a problem, she says. 'It's nothing that bothers me. I'm just aware when it's happening.' And medical examinations have consistently shown Dawn that she is healthy. 'I have to have an examination before I do filming of any sort,' she explains. 'I don't have high blood pressure or any heart problems or anything like that.'

Despite her good health, Dawn has come up against medical disapproval based on her size. 'There are so many mixed messages from the medical profession. There's the strange fascist world of the charts you have to fit into in order to get your mortgage or to adopt a child,' she says. Indeed, when Dawn and her husband Lenny Henry wanted to adopt a baby, Dawn's weight was the only issue standing in the way. 'We passed all the criteria. They looked into our marriage, our finances, our suitability as parents,' Dawn explains. 'You have six months of interviews and your life is pretty much investigated in every way, and it's fairly upsetting and invasive.' The couple got through all of that, and their social worker was perfectly happy. 'It was the doctor who felt she could halt the whole procedure purely because of my weight.' According to the charts, Dawn was well outside the weight limit for a woman of her height.

'My own doctor knows the history of my health, and how good it is, and wouldn't have had any issue with it at all. But I had to promise this doctor from the Adoption Agency that I would lose X-stone in order to fit into their strange, narrow chart on the wall.' Dawn feels this was a fraudulent thing to do because she had no intention of trying to keep her weight down once the child came to them. But she lost the weight because she wanted to adopt so badly. 'It's perfectly possible to achieve weight loss if that's what you're set on, and I did it in order to achieve this child. But it was a lie.' Surely, she says, offering a child the chance to grow up in a household where weight isn't an issue should be seen as a wonderful bonus. 'Personally I think that's something to celebrate. But somehow having a fat mum is not okay.'

Dawn is a successful television and screen actress and comedienne, and one of Britain's best-loved stars. However, even within her own industry she feels marginalised. In fact, she says her size is generally only a disadvantage for her in her professional life. 'I think it seriously hinders my professional opportunities, which is why, very early on, I made the decision to write virtually everything I'm in. That way I don't lessen my scope. I want a diverse career and I don't want anybody to tell me I can't do something because of my shape.' When she first left college Dawn became involved with The Comic Strip, and made about 30 films with them. 'In every single one of those films I played whatever the female role was, whether it was a whore or a prime minister's wife or a bank manager. My size made no difference whatsoever.'

When she left The Comic Strip, however, entering the 'real world' was a huge shock. Since then, she says, she is either typecast or simply not considered for certain roles. 'I'm excluded from being the love interest at the centre of a drama, because it's just not done. To be a deliciously desired woman is not open to me.' And frankly, she says, on the rare occasion she gets a scripts sent to her, the role is usually the same. 'It will always be a fat person, or a girl with eating problems or low self-esteem,' she explains. 'That equals fat. So I know perfectly well where I belong.'

Dawn now develops a variety of projects though the company she runs with partner Jennifer Saunders, and so is able to create a variety of interesting roles for herself. 'If I was an actress who sat by the phone waiting for offers to come, I wouldn't get them. That is a real shame,' she says. 'And that means there's a whole group of bigger actresses who don't get a look-in unless the part requires a big woman.' She also points out that often, when she's described in a review or article, she's not just called Dawn French. 'I'm called roly-poly Dawn French or fat and funny Dawn French or cuddly Dawn French. It doesn't hurt me, but I find it bizarre. I just can't understand why my shape comes before my name. It's very odd.'

Despite her high profile, Dawn feels uncomfortable being described as a spokesperson on behalf of fat people. 'I'm simply not that. I might be an example of a fat person who is successful in their career, and therefore it befalls me to be a spokeswoman,' she says. 'But I don't want to do that any more. I just want to get on with the work that I do, and hope that, with any luck, I'm just a living example.' In fact, she says, being called a role model is in a way patronising. It suggests, she feels, that she's been very brave forging ahead with her career, despite her awful shape. 'And I won't have that. I would rather be respected for the work I do than the size I am.' Dawn French is just incredibly down-to-earth. While she acknowledges there are problems out there for overweight people, she simply tries to work her way through them. When she got fed up with not being able to find clothes to fit her, for example, she decided to start her own plus-size clothes shop, 1647 (so-called because 47 per cent of women are size 16 and over). 'I'm not that interested in fashion actually, but I feel that if you can't get dressed in the morning, if you can't have that simple freedom, how can you be confident about the rest of the day?' There should be a variety of clothes on offer to people of all shapes and sizes, so everyone can make a choice. 'That's the first empowering thing, and then you can get on with whatever you're going to do with your life. That's a huge step,' she says, 'and it's only clothes, but it makes a very big difference.

'We have women who come into the shop, damaged women,

who have been excluded from the experience of shopping for clothes for so many years that they weep when they find some trousers that fit them. Now, what have we done to make that the case?' Dawn asks. As well as largely being ostracised by the fashion industry, Dawn feels women who reach this point have probably never had a positive influence, like her father, in their lives.

'They didn't have this moment where someone said, "You're worth it, and don't let anyone tell you you're not. Don't be invisible and don't be afraid, and don't think you're discountable, because you're not". And I utterly believe that of myself and of every other big woman I come across. You know,' she says, 'the beauty very often is breathtaking. And yet these women have been taught to loathe themselves, and I think that's a huge tyranny.'

However, Dawn believes things are, at last, really starting to change. 'We're in the middle of a fantastic, positive revolution,' she says. 'There's lots of young, angry, big girls who've got plenty to say, who will not settle for no choice and will not be discounted, and that's exactly how it should be.' Dawn even feels that some of these women find her smug and cosy. 'And that's okay. These are proud, fat young women, and that's fine with me,' she smiles.

And proud, vocal women obviously run in Dawn's family. 'My daughter loves to take all her clothes off and look at herself in the mirror. She's six and she's very interested in parts of the body. When anybody comes into the house she has to stick her hand up their blouse,' Dawn laughs. 'I don't know if this is normal. I hope so! Anyway, she was looking in the mirror the other day and she suddenly said, "I hope I get fat soon". There's no answer to that!' Some people might see that as a bit warped, says Dawn. 'But I think it's so great that she can value me as her fat mum, you know, and she doesn't think twice about it. She hopes she'll get bigger because she sees that as a good thing.'

INDEX

INDEX

USEFUL CONTACTS

ALTERNATIVE SIZE
P.O. Box 13882
Fulham
London
SW6 4ZT
Tel: 0171 731 7436
www.larger.com

THE EATING DISORDERS
ASSOCIATION
1st Floor Wensum House
103 Prince of Wales Road
Norwich
Norfolk
NR1 1DW
Tel: 01603 619 090
www.gurney.org.uk/eda/

SLIMMING WORLD
Class Enquiry Line:
01773 521111
www.info@slimming-world.co.uk

1647
69 Gloucester Avenue
London
NW1 8LD

BIG, BOLD & BEAUTIFUL –
MAIL ORDER
1263 Bay Street
Toronto, Ontario
Canada
M5R 2C1
Tel: 00 1 416 923 4673

NATIONAL ASSOCIATION TO
ADVANCE FAT ACCEPTANCE
P.O. Box 188620
Sacramento, CA 95818
USA
Tel: 00 1 916 558 6880
http:\\naafa.org

RICHARD SIMMONS
P.O Box 5403
Beverly Hills, CA 90209-5403
USA
www.richardsimmons.com